THE BIG
BOOK OF
Resident
Activities

Debbie R. Bera, ADC

The Big Book of Resident Activities is published by HCPro, Inc.

ISBN 978-1-60146-169-8

Debbie R. Bera, ADC, Author
Holly Sox, Reviewer
Adrienne Trivers, Managing Editor
Elizabeth Petersen, Executive Editor
Emily Sheahan, Group Publisher
Shane Katz, Cover Designer
Jackie Diehl Singer, Graphic Artist
Audrey Doyle, Copyeditor
Alison Forman, Proofreader
Darren Kelly, Books Production Supervisor
Susan Darbyshire, Art Director
Jean St. Pierre, Director of Operations

Advice given is general. Readers should consult professional counsel for specific legal, ethical, or clinical questions.

Arrangements can be made for quantity discounts. For more information, contact:

HCPro, Inc.

P.O. Box 1168

Marblehead, MA 01945

Telephone: 800/650-6787 or 781/639-1872

Fax: 781/639-2982

E-mail: *customerservice@hcpro.com*

Visit HCPro at its World Wide Web sites:

www.hcpro.com and *www.hcmarketplace.com*

5/2008

21434

Table of Contents

Chapter 1: Activities in Long-Term Care: CMS Regulations 1

    Determination of Compliance 6

    Surveyor Questions and Interviews 7

    Activities Director Responsibilities 9

    Determination of Compliance 10

    Interpretive Guidelines: Assessment 11

    Interpretive Guidelines: Care Planning 11

    Investigative Protocol 12

Chapter 2: Activity Care Plans 21

Chapter 3: Holidays, Birthdays, Special Events, and Themed Activities 47

    Activity: '50s Day 49

    Activity: Annual King and Queen of Hearts Dance 51

    Activity: Annual Sweetheart Dinner 54

    Activity: Back-to-School Week (August or September Event) 57

    Activity: Beach/Hawaiian Day 61

    Activity: Birthday Party 65

    Activity: Camping Week (or Day) 67

    Activity: Chinese New Year Theme Day 70

    Activity: Christmas Charades 73

    Activity: Cruise Week 75

    Activity: Dairy Days Theme Week (June) 78

    Activity: Folk Fair 83

    Activity: Gay '90s Luncheon 86

    Activity: Grandparents' Day Party 88

    Activity: Halloween Party 90

    Activity: Mardi Gras Theme Day 93

    Activity: Mexican Fiesta Day 96

    Activity: New Year's Celebration 99

    Activity: President's Day Silhouettes 101

    Activity: Resident Academy Awards 103

    Activity: Senior Prom 105

    Activity: Spring Fling Party/Social 107

    Activity: St. Patrick's Day Party/Social 109

Activity: Thanksgiving Blessings 111

Activity: Thanksgiving Social 113

Activity: Wedding Week 115

Activity: Western Day 118

Activity: Wine and Cheese Tasting 121

Activity: Winter Charades 122

Activity: Winter Olympics Week 124

**Chapter 4: Activities for Residents with Dementia, Alzheimer's,
and Behavioral Issues** **127**

Stages of Dementia 127

Specialized Dementia Programming and Multisensory Rooms 131

Activity: ABC Game 135

Activity: Afternoon Multisensory Room Program 138

Activity: Big Ball Fun 141

Activity: Bubble Mania 143

Activity: Colors and Shapes Bingo 145

Activity: Creative-Expressive 147

Activity: Creative Writing Group 149

Activity: Dice Game 152

Activity: Dusterball 154

Activity: Evening Dementia Program 156

Activity: Five Alive 159

Activity: Folded Paper Paintings 162

Activity: Grandma's Kitchen on a Cart 165

Activity: Hands Alive 168

Activity: Hidden Treasures Sensory 170

Activity: Match Game 172

Activity: Memory Matching 174

Activity: Morning Wakeup Sensory Program 176

Activity: Music with Movement Program for the Memory/Sensory Program 178

Activity: Name Five 181

Activity: Noodle Ball 183

Activity: Noodle Exercise 186

Activity: Object Identification 189

Activity: Parachute Fun 191

Activity: Pet Therapy/Pet Visits 193

Activity: Picture Postcard Memories 195

Activity: Recreational Programs 197

Activity: Relaxation Music with Movement for Sensory Program 199

Activity: Rice Bag Sensory 202

Activity: Rise and Shine 205

Activity: Seashell Sensory 208

Activity: Sensory Stimulation Programs 210

Activity: Sorting Box 213

Activity: Sound Effects Sensory 215

Activity: Themed Sensory Kits 217

Activity: Therapeutic Massage 220

**Chapter 5: Adapting and Modifying Activities to Accommodate
Individual Resident Needs** **223**

Common Impairments and Adaptations/Intervention 225

Chapters 6: Activities for Younger Residents and Short-Term Stay Residents **229**

Activity: Daily Crossword or Trivia 232

Activity: Library Cart 234

Activity: Martial Arts/Adapted Tae Kwon Do 236

Activity: Pilates 241

Activity: Social Time 246

Activity: Tai Chi 248

Activity: Walking Club 252

Activity: Weekend Trivia 254

Activity: Welcome Initiative 256

Activity: Yoga 258

Chapter 7: Activities for Men **263**

Activity: 6,5,4 Dice Game 265

Activity: Men's Card Club 268

Activity: Men's Club Breakfast/Luncheon 270

Activity: Men's Club Grill-Out or Picnic 272

Activity: Men's Gathering/Coffee and Gab Session 274

Activity: Romeo Club 276

Activity: Turkey Shoot 278

Chapter 8: Activities for Women **281**

Activity: Cooking Club 283

Activity: Devotional/Prayer Group 285

Activity: Fashion Show 287

Activity: Fondue Party/Social 289

Activity: Gardening Club 298

Activity: Red Hat Society 301

Activity: Scrapbooking 304

Activity: Spa Day 307

Activity: Tea Social/Gourmet Coffee Social 309

Chapter 9: Activities for Bariatric Residents **311**

Activity: Bariatric Ball Exercise 314

Activity: Bariatric Cooking Class 318

Activity: Bariatric Exercise 324

Chapter 10: One-on-One Activities **329**

Activity: Memories 332

Activity: Morning Stretch 334

Chapter 11: The Activities Calendar **337**

Chapter 12: Involving Residents and Family Members in Activities **343**

Activity: Annual Picnic 345

Activity: Comfort Cart 347

Activity: Craft and Bake Sale 349

Activity: Facility Dog Show 352

Activity: Father's Day Brunch 354

Activity: Fun Fair 356

Activity: Memorial Service 358

Activity: Mother's Day Tea Social 360

Activity: Outdoor Campfire Night 362

Activity: Resident/Family Christmas Tea Social 364

Activity: Wishing Well 366

Chapter 1

Activities in Long-Term Care: CMS Regulations

One reason the Centers for Medicare & Medicaid Services (CMS) rewrote the guidelines is that CMS is a strong supporter of culture change as it applies to resident-centered care. This means creating a home-like environment for residents of long-term care facilities; in essence, ensuring that these facilities look the way we would want them to look if we were residing in them.

Another reason was to improve the quality of life for individuals residing in long-term care facilities. *Quality of life* can be a subjective term, but generally you can improve a resident's quality of life by enhancing his or her self-esteem and dignity. Each resident's involvement in daily life should be meaningful. Activities are meaningful when they reflect a person's interests and lifestyle, when they are enjoyable to the person, when they help the person to feel useful, and when they provide the person with a sense of belonging. Residents themselves indicate that a lack of activities in long-term care facilities contributes to their feeling of having no sense of purpose.

"Activities" refer to any endeavor, other than routine activities of daily living (ADLs), in which a resident participates that is intended to enhance the resident's sense of well-being and promote or enhance his or her physical, cognitive/intellectual, spiritual, social, and emotional health. These include, but are not limited to, activities that promote:

- Self-esteem

- Pleasure

- Comfort

- Education

- Creativity

- Success

- Independence

Two F tags are specific to activities. CMS wrote these F tags in 1989 and implemented them in 1990 to teach long-term care facilities the importance of quality activities to residents' well-being. They are F248, a key outcome tag within Quality of Life; and F249, which concerns the presence within the facility of an activities director who is qualified to serve in that role. Although the codes have not changed, the Interpretive Guidelines have changed, and became effective June 1, 2006. This means surveyors are looking at activities in a new light, using the new investigative protocol during the survey process. OBRA '87 is used as a basis to support culture change in long-term care as well as to support the investigative guidelines requiring an interdisciplinary approach toward meeting the leisure and psychosocial needs of those we serve in long-term care.

The following is a brief overview of the new Federal Interpretive Guidelines for F248 and F249:

- Resident outcomes are a key feature of determining whether a facility's activities program is adequate for each resident, because the regulation specifies that activities be individualized for each resident.

- The guidelines mandate that the facility considers each resident's varying interests so that the mere development of a program is not sufficient for compliance. In other words, a facility cannot simply place its residents into whatever activities are available. Instead, the facility must individualize activities according to each resident's interests, to enhance his or her well-being.

- Residents may be unable to pursue prior interests unless the facility makes an effort to provide adaptations or assistance. The facility should realize that residents can also develop new interests.

- "One-to-one programming" refers to programming provided to residents who will not, or cannot, effectively plan their own activity pursuits, or to residents who need specialized or extended programs to enhance their overall daily routine and activity pursuits.

- "Person-appropriate" activities refer to the idea that each resident has a personal identity and history that includes much more than just his or her medical illnesses or functional impairments, and that activities should be as relevant as possible to the specific needs, interests, culture, background, and so on of the individual for whom they are developed. Such activities reflect what the resident likes and responds to. "Person-appropriate" replaces "age-appropriate," as carrying a doll can be appropriate for some residents.

- "Program of activities" includes a combination of large and small groups, a one-to-one program, and self-directed activities; it also includes a system that supports the development, implementation, and evaluation of the activities provided to the residents in the facility. It does not mean that every facility needs to offer every type of activity; rather, the facility should base its range of programming types on the interests of its residents. Surveyors will evaluate a facility's program to determine whether it accommodates the residents who live there.

- The program of activities should allow for spontaneous changes if residents desire. The key is resident choice.

- Reality orientation and large group activities that include residents of different levels of strengths and needs are not recommended.

- The activity assessment (which will be looked at extensively) needs to be specific enough for the facility to develop a care plan that meets its residents' interests, and for the facility to understand what specific adaptations and assistance are needed. Surveyors will evaluate the assessment and care plan to see whether activities are individualized for each resident. They will determine whether the care plan reflects what is actually occurring at the facility, and whether they see it occurring.

- The interdisciplinary team should take into account various components of residents' schedules to optimize resident choice to the greatest extent possible (i.e., individualize each resident's schedule).

- If a resident needs assistance to travel to locations where activities are taking place in the building, the facility needs to provide the necessary transportation both to and from these activities, as well as any special clothing that may be needed. The various departments need to work together on care planning to make sure residents arrive at their preferred activities on time. Surveyors will determine whether needed assistance is provided.

- The facility should provide needed supplies and equipment according to each resident's care plan (e.g., eyeglasses, hearing aids, etc.), to optimize their participation. Surveyors will determine whether needed supplies and equipment are provided.

- The facility should adapt its activities to accommodate a particular resident's change in functioning to the greatest degree possible. Such adaptations can include special equipment, special techniques used to interact with the resident, and changes to the environment where such activities are taking place.

- Residents are not required to attend activities. However, the facility should determine what it needs to do to help residents pursue independent leisure interests and to keep residents informed about activities in the facility, as well as periodically asking residents if they wish to attend anything. The facility needs to determine whether the resident's choices reflect a lifelong pattern and whether the resident is content with his or her choices.

- Facilities should take into account a resident's pattern of behavioral symptoms and activities prior to when such symptoms usually present themselves. This is important because once a behavior escalates activities may be less effective or may cause further stress. The facility should try to individualize its approach toward residents who appear distressed or who exhibit a pattern of aggressive or anxious behavior. Approaches need to be specific enough that the staff can employ them routinely.

- Specific interventions must be individualized, even when different individuals display similar behavior (i.e., no "canned" care plans).

- Surveyors will ask residents for their opinion of the activities the facility offers, whether the activities occur as scheduled, whether they are satisfied that these activities meet their preferences, and whether the environment in which the activities take place poses any barriers.

- Surveyors will determine whether the facility found out about a resident's previous activities, choices, preferences, and need for adaptation, and what the records indicate.

- Surveyors will determine whether residents participated in the development of their care plan.

- Surveyors will determine whether the facility periodically reviews the care plan with its residents and makes needed changes.

The new guidelines have far-reaching effects into all other departments within the facility. For example, some medications, such as diuretics, or conditions, such as pain and incontinence, may affect resident participation in activities. Therefore, additional steps may be needed to facilitate resident participation. Some of these steps include:

- Changing the timing of medications, to the greatest extent possible if not contraindicated, so that the resident can participate and remain at a scheduled activity.

- Modifying when pain meds are administered to allow such meds to take effect prior to an activity a resident enjoys.

- Considering accommodations in schedules, supplies, and timing to optimize residents' ability to participate in their activities of choice. This can include altering a therapy or bath schedule if a desired activity occurs at the same time; helping a resident to get to and participate in desired activities; providing supplies for activities; and providing assistance as needed during weekends, nights, holidays, or when the activities staff is unavailable.

The interpretive guidelines specifically state that all staff members are responsible for each resident's quality of life. This means the perception of what constitutes "activities" needs to change. Just because the activities staff is not in the building does not mean that activities do not occur. Activities are often led by volunteers, and even by residents. CMS expects that all staff members are responsible for providing activities. This has always been in the code; now CMS is enforcing it.

F248: "The facility must provide for an ongoing program of activities designed to meet, in accordance with the comprehensive assessment, the interests and the physical, mental, and psychosocial well-being of each resident."

This regulatory language includes the specific term "the facility," which indicates that the provision of activities is not the duty of the Activities Department, but rather is the duty of the facility as a whole.

It is not possible for a few people in an Activities Department to be able to provide individualized activities for the facility's entire population; therefore, the writers of the regulation chose to make it the responsibility of the facility as a whole to fulfill this important mandate of the OBRA '87 law.

The intent is for the facility to identify each resident's interests and needs; toward that end, the facility should involve each resident in an ongoing program of activities that is designed to appeal to his or her interests and to enhance the resident's highest practicable level of physical, mental, and psychosocial well-being.

Determination of Compliance

A facility is in compliance if it:

- Recognized and assessed residents for preferences, choices, specific conditions, causes and/or problems, needs, and behaviors

- Defined and implemented activities in accordance with resident needs and goals

- Monitored and evaluated each resident's response to activity interventions

- Revised its approaches toward activities as appropriate

- Determined compliance separately for each resident sampled

- Individualized activity interventions to each resident's needs and preferences

- Provided necessary adaptations to facilitate residents' participation

A facility might be in noncompliance if:

- Off-campus activities are planned only for more independent residents due to lack of staff members

- No activities are available when the Activities Department staff is not there (e.g., on weekends), and residents complain of having nothing to do

- The facility places residents into large group activities that are not geared toward their individual interests and/or capabilities, and residents who are present at these activities are routinely trying to leave the room or are disengaged and sleeping, yelling, or otherwise expressing discomfort

- Residents who are confined to their rooms complain of having nothing to do, activity staff members say they are too busy to get to everyone, and/or no other departments help with activities for these residents

- Residents do not receive the adaptations they need to participate in individualized activities

- Planned activities are not conducted or are not designed to meet the needs of the care plan

- Residents are not dressed, out of bed, and ready to attend activities in which they want to participate

- The staff does not coordinate schedules of medication and therapies, resulting in residents being unable to attend programs of interest

There are other potential tags for additional investigation if a citation is made in F248 or F249. Deficiencies at F248 are most likely to have psychosocial outcomes. Most citations will fall at Level 2 or 3.

Surveyor Questions and Interviews

The surveyors will be interviewing certified nursing assistants about how they provide activities to residents and their role in ensuring that residents are out of bed, dressed, and ready to participate in their chosen activities. Some of the questions surveyors may ask include:

- How do you help individual residents participate in activities?

- What is your role in activities conducted by the Activities Department?

- Do you provide any activities when the activities staff is not present?

- How and when do you assist residents who are confined to their room with setup/ positioning, and so on to allow for independent activity?

The surveyors also will interview the social services staff. Some questions they may ask include:

- How do you help residents participate in activities?

- What is your role in ensuring that residents are able to attend activities such as plays? (For example, is it your responsibility to procure the equipment and funds necessary to offer such activities?)

In addition, the surveyors will interview nurses at your facility. They may ask such questions as:

- How do you help each resident to participate in his or her chosen activities?

- How do you coordinate residents' schedules of ADLs, medications, and therapies so that they can participate in their chosen activities?

- What does the nursing staff provide during off-hours and for residents who cannot attend group activities?

The housekeeping, maintenance, dietary, and nutrition staffs all can provide positive social interactions, which raises residents' self-esteem and in turn has a positive effect on their quality of life. All of the facility's staff members should interact with residents, even in passing—for example, by complimenting how they look, commenting on the weather, and reassuring anxious residents. The staff should also take the time to ensure that residents are not bored, but rather that they have something to do, ensuring that whatever diversion they provide to a resident is within that resident's abilities; for example, they should not give a magazine to someone who cannot turn the pages.

Surveyors will determine whether staff members know what they are supposed to do according to the care plan and whether they are doing it. Surveyors also will determine whether staff members from different departments are working as a team to ensure that residents can participate in their activities of choice.

F249: The activities program must be directed by a qualified professional who:
(i)   Is a qualified therapeutic recreation specialist or an activities professional who:

(A)   Is licensed or registered, if applicable, by the state in which he or she is practicing; and

(B)   Is eligible for certification as a therapeutic recreation specialist or as an activities professional by a recognized accrediting body on or after October 1, 1990; or

(ii)   Has two years of experience in a social or recreational program within the past five years, one of which was full-time in a patient activities program in a healthcare setting; or

(iii)   Is a qualified occupational therapist or occupational therapy assistant; or

(iv)   Has completed a training course approved by the state.

The intent is to ensure that a facility's activities program is directed by a qualified professional, and that the activities director remains eligible for this position by keeping up with whatever the state requires. If the state requires the director to have a license or be certified, the director must keep his or her status current.

F249 is an absolute requirement, which means that if a facility fails to meet the regulatory language in F249, the facility is cited, regardless of whether there are outcomes to its residents.

Activities Director Responsibilities

The activities director is responsible for the program, its compliance with the regulatory mandates in F248, and its implementation by the staff and volunteers who are conducting aspects of the program; for example, those individuals know what to do, they furnish residents with supplies, equipment, and sufficient space, and so on. The director's responsibilities also include:

- Directing the development, implementation, supervision, and ongoing evaluation of the activities program

- Completing or delegating the completion of the activities component of the comprehensive assessment

- Contributing to, directing, or delegating the contribution to the goals of the comprehensive care plan

"Ongoing evaluation" means:

- Determining whether the program as a whole includes offerings that meet resident preferences and needs

- Determining whether changes are needed, such as new seasonal programs for certain times of the year

- Assessing whether the program includes activities for different interests and needs, for residents who are unable to participate in group offerings, for residents who want activities in the evenings and on weekends, and so on

The director is responsible for the activities component of each resident's assessment. The director needs to contribute to the activities component of the comprehensive care plan information regarding what individualized activities the resident will be participating in, and what the resident will need in order to participate. The interdisciplinary team should work together to ensure that the resident receives any necessary transportation and adaptation to allow participation. This is the facility's responsibility, to ensure that the resident's care plan is implemented.

"Directing the program" means scheduling activities to meet residents' needs. This involves more than merely producing a monthly calendar. It includes ensuring that activity interventions for all residents can occur; for example, activities have assigned space, essential supplies, and someone to lead or facilitate them.

Monitoring resident responses may be done in part by those staff members who are conducting the activity. The director needs to remain informed of resident responses to activities to determine whether changes are needed in any of the activity offerings.

The director is also responsible for taking the information gathered regarding needed changes and actually making those changes to the activity program offerings.

Determination of Compliance

A facility is in compliance if it has employed a qualified activities director who:

- Has developed an activities program that meets the interests of residents

- Ensures that the activities component of the comprehensive assessment is completed for every resident and contributes to care plan goals

- Monitors residents' responses to interventions and makes necessary changes to care plans and/or to the program offerings

Noncompliance for F249

Noncompliance may include:

- Lack of a qualified activities director

- Lack of direction for planning, scheduling, implementing, monitoring, and revising the activities program

- Lack of monitoring the response of residents to modify care plans as needed

The severity for a deficiency at F249 is based on the effect or potential for harm to the resident. After a deficiency is cited at F249, the severity and scope that are selected *do* need to consider outcomes and potential outcomes to residents.

Interpretive Guidelines: Assessment

The information from the assessment needs to be specific enough for the facility to develop a care plan to meet residents' interests, and to be able to understand what specific adaptation and assistance are required.

Some residents are capable of self-structuring their day, and this needs to be noted in their assessment and identified on their plan of care. In assessing each resident, the staff should note what the resident prefers, what adaptations are needed, and what the resident's lifelong interests, spirituality, goals, life roles, skills, abilities, and needs are.

Interpretive Guidelines: Care Planning

Information from the individualized assessment is used to develop the activities components of the comprehensive care plan. Objectives should be measurable and should focus on the resident's desired outcomes. All relevant departments collaborate—not just the Activities Department. Individualized interventions are based on an assessment of each resident's history, preferences, strengths, and needs. Many activities can be adapted to accommodate a particular resident's change in functioning. The facility should be aware of the range of adaptations it can make to assist residents in participating in their activities of choice. It is important to identify whether the resident has issues for which the staff should provide adaptations. Types of impairments that might require adaptations include visual, hearing, physical, and cognitive. Some adaptations employ special equipment; others involve adapting the environment where activities are taking place. For some residents, the length of the activity may need to change or the steps of the activity may need to be task-segmented into simple steps.

Some residents who have dementia may have a pattern of aggressive or anxious behavior at a similar time each day. The facility should try to individualize its approach to residents with distressed behavior, taking all factors into account. Sometimes a simple diversion may suffice, such as engaging the resident in a quiet and pleasant conversation, offering a drink or snack, or asking the resident to help with something. These staff interactions should be part of the resident's care plan and should be specific for the staff to use them routinely.

Investigative Protocol

Surveyors evaluate the ongoing program of activities to determine whether it accommodates the residents who live at the facility. Surveyors look at the assessment and care plan to see whether preferences and needs are taken into account, any necessary adaptive equipment is used, timely transportation is provided if needed, and available activities are compatible with residents' interests, needs, and abilities. They also look to see whether any significant changes have occurred in activity patterns. They determine whether the residents' activities-related care plan:

- Includes participation of the resident (if able) or the resident's representative

- Considers a continuation of life roles, consistent with preferences and functional capacity, and encourages and supports the development of new interests, hobbies, and skills

- Identifies interventions that include activities in the community, if appropriate, and includes needed adaptations that address resident conditions and issues affecting activity participation

- Identifies how the facility will provide activities to help residents reach their goal(s), as well as who is responsible for implementing various interventions

Surveyors also observe activities to see whether residents are engaged in these activities—that is, whether residents are looking at staff and listening to what is being said, smiling, or responding to the activities in some other way. They also observe to see whether residents are disengaged—that is, whether residents are looking down, sleeping, or attempting to leave the room. If a resident is doing this, surveyors watch to see what the staff will do.

Figure 1.1	ACTIVITY INTERVIEW ASSESSMENT

	Type of Assessment:
Resident Name:	**Admission** **Quarterly**
Wing/Unit & Room Number:	**Annual** **Significant change**
Medical Record Number:	**Other: (specify)**
Date of Assessment:	**Participation in Assessment:**
Staff Signature & Date:	Resident Family Other staff Chart/notes
	Personal observations of staff completing assessment

Hearing/ability to hear:

Adequate – no difficulty in normal conversation, social interaction, listening to TV

Minimal difficulty – difficulty in some environments (e.g., when spoken to softly or when setting is noisy)

Moderate difficulty – speaker has to increase volume and speak distinctly

Highly impaired – absence of useful hearing

Uses hearing aide or appliance: Yes/No   Type:

Speech clarity:

Clear speech – distinct intelligible words

Unclear speech – slurred or mumbled words

No speech – absence of spoken words

Makes self understood:

Understood

Usually understood – difficulty communicating some words or finishing thoughts, but is able if prompted or given time

Sometimes understood – ability is limited to making concrete requests

Rarely/never understood

Ability to understand others:

Understands – clear comprehension

Usually understands – misses some part/intent of message, but comprehends most conversations

Sometimes understands – responds adequately to simple, direct communication only

Rarely/never understands

Figure 1.1

ACTIVITY INTERVIEW ASSESSMENT (cont.)

Vision:

Adequate – sees fine detail, including regular print in newspapers/books

Impaired – sees large print, but not regular print in newspapers/books

Moderately impaired – limited vision; not able to see newspaper headlines but can identify objects

Highly impaired – object identification in question, but eyes appear to follow objects

Severely impaired – no vision or sees only light, colors, or shapes; eyes do not appear to follow objects

Wears glasses: Yes/No   Uses magnifying glass: Yes/No

Mental status:

Short-term memory (seems or appears to recall after five minutes)

Memory okay

Memory problem

Long-term memory (seems or appears to recall long past memories)

Memory okay

Memory problem

Memory/recall ability Circle all that he or she can normally recall

Current season   Location of room

Staff names and faces   That he or she is in a nursing home

None of the above

Attention span

Short   Average   Long   Easily distracted   Focuses well   Not able to focus   Poor

Cognitive skills for daily decision-making:

Independent – decision consistent/reasonable

Modified independence – some difficulty in new situations

Moderately impaired – decisions poor; cues/supervision required

Severely impaired – never/rarely makes decisions

Psychosocial/mood:

Little interest or pleasure in doing things

Feeling down, depressed, or hopeless

Social in nature and enthusiastic

Supportive family/friends

Appears to have good coping skills

Figure 1.2

ACTIVITY PROGRESS NOTE

Resident:	Room #:	Medical record #:	Date:

Purpose for note:

❑ Annual review ❑ Quarterly review ❑ Significant change ❑ Other:

> Visit/group/independent activity enjoyed/pursued:

MDS Activity Pursuit patterns section review:

❑ MDS reviewed, and no changes were made to the Activity Pursuit section.

❑ MDS reviewed, and the changes made to the Activity Pursuit section include:

Attendance/participation summary (refer to activity flow sheets/attendance sheets):

Attended on: ❑ Own ❑ Needs assistance ❑ Wheelchair ❑ Cane
❑ Wheeled walker ❑ Walker ❑ Tilt-back chair ❑ Walks
❑ Other:_____

Describe resident's participation in/response to activities (group, 1:1 visits, and/or individual):

Activity plan review:

Resident's activity-related problem(s) (include needs, concerns, and/or strengths)

❑ Remain appropriate/current ❑ Will be retained

Detail problem changes:_____

_____

Figure 1.2

ACTIVITY PROGRESS NOTE (cont.)

❏ Have been resolved/changed   ❏ Will be revised
❏ New problems have emerged

Progress toward resident's activity plan goals(s):
 ❏ Surpassed goal   ❏ Goal will be increased

Detail goal changes: _____

_____

 ❏ Met goal   ❏ Goal will be decreased

 ❏ Did not meet goal   ❏ Goal will be retained

 ❏ Goal unsuitable   ❏ Goal will be revised

Appropriateness of activity interventions:

 ❏ Interventions remain effective

Detail intervention changes:_____

_____

 ❏ Interventions are partially effective

 ❏ Interventions will be revised

Additional comments:

Signature: _____ Title/credentials: _____

Figure 1.3

QUARTERLY ACTIVITY RESPONSE REVIEW

Quarterly Activity Response Review

Resident Name: _____   Medical Record Number: _____

Circle **ALL** noted responses/involvement that the resident offers. Define areas as specified.

Annual **Dates:**	**1st Quarter** **Dates:**
Physical abilities: Stable/Declined/Improved Define: Can complete a single-step command: Yes/No Provide example:	Physical abilities: Stable/Declined/Improved Define: Can complete a single-step command: Yes/No Provide example:
Displays simple large motor skills: Yes/No Can complete a multistep command: Yes/No Provide example:	Displays simple large motor skills: Yes/No Can complete a multistep command: Yes/No Provide example:
Mood: Stable/Variable/Declined/Improved Define:	Mood: Stable/Variable/Declined/Improved Define:
Behaviors: None/Stable/Improved/Declined Define: Displays anxiety/restlessness at activities: Yes/No Define behavior:	Behaviors: None/Stable/Improved/Declined Define: Displays anxiety/restlessness at activities: Yes/No Define behavior:
Displays repetitive behavior: Yes/No Define behavior:	Displays repetitive behavior: Yes/No Define behavior:
Cognition: Stable/Improved/Declined Define:	Cognition: Stable/Improved/Declined Define:
Has a limited attention span: Yes/No Exhibited by: Loss of attention span after _____ min. Reestablishes attention to activity with prompting: Yes/No Remains alert and attentive/attention span intact: Yes/No Falls asleep during activities: Yes/No Needs verbal cues to complete tasks: Yes/No Needs visual cues to complete tasks: Yes/No Needs direct physical guidance/hand-over-hand: Yes/No	Has a limited attention span: Yes/No Exhibited by: Loss of attention span after _____ min. Reestablishes attention to activity with prompting: Yes/No Remains alert and attentive/attention span intact: Yes/No Falls asleep during activities: Yes/No Needs verbal cues to complete tasks: Yes/No Needs visual cues to complete tasks: Yes/No Needs direct physical guidance/hand-over-hand: Yes/No

Social interaction/communication abilities:

1 – 2-word response	Nonverbal
Unrelated conversation	Appropriate sentences
Facial expressions	Gestures
Body posture change	Answers simple question

Displays social/interactive skills
Displays physical demonstration of understanding
Displays long-term memory skills
Displays short-term memory skills
Displays congenial verbal responses
Comments:

Social interaction/communication abilities:

1 – 2-word response	Nonverbal
Unrelated conversation	Appropriate sentences
Facial expressions	Gestures
Body posture change	Answers simple question

Displays social/interactive skills
Displays physical demonstration of understanding
Displays long-term memory skills
Displays short-term memory skills
Displays congenial verbal responses
Comments:

Most successful interventions/favorite activities: Most successful interventions/favorite activities:

Figure 1.3

QUARTERLY ACTIVITY RESPONSE REVIEW (cont.)

Quarterly Activity Response Review

Resident Name: _____   Medical Record Number: _____

Circle **ALL** noted responses/involvement that the resident offers. Define areas as specified.

2nd Quarter　　　　**Dates:**	**3rd Quarter**　　　　**Dates:**
Physical abilities: Stable/Declined/Improved Define:	Physical abilities: Stable/Declined/Improved Define:
Can complete a single-step command: Yes/No Provide example:	Can complete a single-step command: Yes/No Provide example:
Can complete a multistep command: Yes/No Provide example:	Can complete a multistep command: Yes/No Provide example:
Displays simple large motor skills: Yes/No Mood: Stable/Variable/Declined/Improved Define:	Displays simple large motor skills: Yes/No Mood: Stable/Variable/Declined/Improved Define:
Behaviors: None/Stable/Improved/Declined Define:	Behaviors: None/Stable/Improved/Declined Define:
Displays anxiety/restlessness at activities: Yes/No Define behavior:	Displays anxiety/restlessness at activities: Yes/No Define behavior:
Displays repetitive behavior: Yes/No Define behavior:	Displays repetitive behavior: Yes/No Define behavior:
Cognition: Stable/Improved/Declined Define:	Cognition: Stable/Improved/Declined Define:
Has a limited attention span: Yes/No Exhibited by:	Has a limited attention span: Yes/No Exhibited by:
Loss of attention span after _____ min.	Loss of attention span after _____ min.
Reestablishes attention to activity with prompting: Yes/No	Reestablishes attention to activity with prompting: Yes/No
Remains alert and attentive/attention span intact: Yes/No	Remains alert and attentive/attention span intact: Yes/No
Falls asleep during activities: Yes/No	Falls asleep during activities: Yes/No
Needs verbal cues to complete tasks: Yes/No	Needs verbal cues to complete tasks: Yes/No
Needs visual cues to complete tasks: Yes/No	Needs visual cues to complete tasks: Yes/No
Needs direct physical guidance/hand-over-hand: Yes/No	Needs direct physical guidance/hand-over-hand: Yes/No
Social interaction/communication abilities:	Social interaction/communication abilities:
1 – 2-word response　　　　Nonverbal	1 – 2-word response　　　　Nonverbal
Unrelated conversation　　　Appropriate sentences	Unrelated conversation　　　Appropriate sentences
Facial expressions　　　　　Gestures	Facial expressions　　　　　Gestures
Body posture change　　　　Answers simple question	Body posture change　　　　Answers simple question
Displays social/interactive skills	Displays social/interactive skills
Displays physical demonstration of understanding	Displays physical demonstration of understanding
Displays long-term memory skills	Displays long-term memory skills
Displays short-term memory skills	Displays short-term memory skills
Displays congenial verbal responses	Displays congenial verbal responses
Comments:	Comments:
Most successful interventions/favorite activities:	Most successful interventions/favorite activities:

Chapter 2

Activity Care Plans

Once a comprehensive activity assessment and Minimum Data Set (MDS) have been completed, it is time to develop an individualized care plan based on the assessment and MDS. Each activity care plan should be resident-focused. "I Care Plans" help to keep the plan of care resident-centered, as they are stated from the residents' point of view. Both the Centers for Medicare & Medicaid Services and the culture change movement recognize "I Care Plans" as a vehicle for moving toward resident-centered care.

A care plan should:

- Be specific enough that it identifies the resident for whom it was developed

- Take into account what resident outcomes you hope to achieve

- Identify the resident's varying interests, including one-on-one activities, small groups, large groups, and independent activity interests

- Include any necessary assistance, adaptations to facilitate the resident's participation, or assistive devices to enable the resident to pursue his or her leisure interests and to optimize his or her participation

- Recognize the resident's needs, interests, preferences, desires, choices, specific conditions, and causes so that the resident can be fully engaged to the best of his or her ability within the programming, and to enhance the resident's highest practicable level of physical, mental, and psychosocial well-being

- Include a way to monitor and evaluate the resident's responses

- Include resident behavior that negatively impacts activities, along with activity interventions that may help to reduce such behavior

- Ensure that approaches for dealing with behavior symptoms are specific enough that all staff members can employ them routinely

- Individualize specific interventions even when different residents display similar behaviors

- Include the resident's past life activities, choices, and preferences

- Include all staff members who play a role in the provision of leisure pursuits for the resident

- Include the resident in the development of his or her care plan to the extent possible

Once an activity care plan is devised, it needs to be routinely reviewed, modified, and revised according to the resident's needs, just as the activity assessment needs to be. The best care plans come from a very thorough assessment of each resident, and from observations made during the resident's participation in activities. Ongoing assessments are based on observations made during interventions/programming. That makes it important for activity professionals to be directly involved in the provision of the activities and not to rely solely on the observations of other staff members.

Short-Term Stay ACTIVITY CARE PLAN			Resident Name:	Room:	Medical Record #:	
Date written:	#1	I expect to have a short-term stay at this facility for rehab. I am able to self-structure my own day and prefer independent leisure pursuits. I have a supportive family. I plan to be here for two weeks and I will focus on therapy while here, but may attend some activities.	I will participate in preferred independent leisure pursuits of TV, reading, word searches, and crafts during my stay through: I will interact with my family via daily visits and with others who are also in therapy on a daily basis during my stay through: I will check out autobiographies from the library cart during the weekly volunteer visits during my stay through:	Review activity calendar with me to identify areas of interest. Introduce me to peers with similar interests and abilities, especially those also here for therapy. Stop in to see me to ensure that I am still content with my independent social and recreational contacts. Encourage independent leisure pursuits of interest; target: TV (public TV, game shows, channel 8, British comedies), reading (autobiographies), family visits, word searches, and crafts (crochet, knit). Inform me of groups of potential interest; target: music (country western), bingo, church, rosary, socials, and trivia. Have the volunteer library cart stop by my room weekly during my stay. Include me in the Weekend Trivia packet as I enjoy trivia and word searches that are a part of that.	Discipline: All All All All All All All	Date of review:

Dementia Program ACTIVITY CARE PLAN				Resident Name:	Room:		Medical Record #:	
Date written:	#2	I have trouble remembering, comprehending, and relaxing. I like to be with others socially and to feel connected to other people. I like to feel successful in what I do. I need the staff to help me to divert my energy and attention and to validate my feelings. I need the staff to help me to gain a greater feeling of comfort at the end of the day, as I can become more anxious at that time.	I will engage in independent, relaxing activities in the early evening hours (e.g., listening to radio, watching TV, reading, using the multisensory room) with staff assistance through: I will have positive outcomes of increased responsiveness (responding to questions/stimuli), social displays, and attention span as evidenced by being able to focus on activities/tasks for 20 – 30 minutes, and by a decrease in anxiety and agitation (visual signs of relaxation) during multisensory room and small-group dementia-specific programming through: I will be able to correctly identify objects in pictures 75% of the time, mimic/mirror actions 100% of the time, and complete one- and two-step tasks during small-group dementia-specific programming through:	Introduce yourself and your purpose upon each contact with me. Call me by my name to capture my attention. Encourage me to verbalize/talk about my past interests (e.g., cooking, baking, raising children, and my faith). Encourage visits by my family/others. Place me near peers when I'm out of my room to give me an opportunity for mental and social stimulation. Talk to me about daily events or objects in my surroundings, and provide reminders/reassurance as appropriate during all contact with me. Offer to discuss with me facility happenings, seasons, holidays, simple current events, and familiar people. Provide me with social visits for connection with others throughout the day. Invite, encourage, and help me to attend programs of interest; target: music (polka, hymns, country, old-time, singalongs), special programs, socials, bingo, exercise, church, rosary, Sunshine Group, and Five Alive. Include me in sensory stimulation, Hands Alive, and massage (which I love). Encourage and set up independent activities of interest for me—for example, reading (women's magazines, religious material), TV (news, older programs, country music station), radio (country or relaxing music), and family visits. Ask me for responses that I can provide. Simplify tasks and reduce stimulation if I'm showing difficulty comprehending and feeling too challenged.	Discipline: All All All All All All All All All All			Date of review:	

Dementia Program ACTIVITY CARE PLAN				Resident Name:	Room:	Medical Record #:	
				Emphasize my abilities and accomplishments. Provide verbal and visual cues and direct physical guidance for tasks within my abilities.	All		
				Reminisce with me about my family, and include me in activities that focus more on long-term memory (e.g., reminiscence groups).	All		
				Include me in multisensory room and small-group dementia-specific programming, and target programs that improve memory recall, object identification, reminiscence skills, reasoning skills, completion of one- or two-step tasks, mirroring actions, relaxation, physical engagement, increased awareness of environment, and cognitive thinking skills. Guide me toward quieting, calming activities, especially in the evening hours (evening dementia programming).	All		

Long-Term Stay ACTIVITY CARE PLAN		Resident Name:	Room:	Medical Record #:	
Date written:	#3	I am very social in nature. I have a great sense of humor. I am able to self-structure my own day. I am willing to participate in activities of interest. I enjoy visiting the activities director in her office several times per day. I am forgetful, but that does not impact my ability to pursue leisure interests. I need reminders of groups, and I like assistance even though I am able to self-propel. I am hard of hearing, so speak in a louder tone and make sure I hear the message.	I will continue to self-direct my day with leisure interests on a daily basis through: I will continue to interact with others daily and share my sense of humor with others through: I will take an active role by completing tasks, offering discussion, and socializing with others through: I will continue to visit with the activities director in her office to "shoot the breeze" and collect a hug through:	Encourage my leisure pursuits of interest—for example, TV (news, family programs), socializing, reading (horse/farm magazines, as I had a big farm), phone contacts with family, family visits, the aviary, and making rounds to visit the activities staff. Invite me to and remind me of/ encourage my participation in and assist me as needed to attend programs of interest; target: music (polka, waltz, country, old-time, guitar, as I used to play it in a band), special programs, church, rosary, bingo, recreational games, Romeo Club, dining out, bus rides, and cooking. Ask me direct questions to promote conversation and an active role. Speak directly to me in a louder tone, and repeat messages as needed to be sure I hear correctly. Make sure my hearing aid is in my right ear. Share good jokes with me.	Discipline: All All All All	Date of review:

THE BIG BOOK OF RESIDENT ACTIVITIES

Dementia Program ACTIVITY CARE PLAN			Resident Name:	Room:	Medical Record #:	
Date written:	#4	I have a profound cognitive impairment. I have trouble with comprehension and reasoning. I have a limited attention span, and keeping me physically engaged/involved helps to maintain my attention. I like to be with others socially and to feel connected to other people. I like to feel successful in what I do. At times, I say, "Hey, hey" to get attention when I have a need.	I will increase my attention span by becoming involved in engaging activities that allow me to complete a simple one-step task, answer simple, direct questions, or offer discussion when prompted with each activity/intervention through: I will continue to spend time in social areas and to interact with others upon approach daily through: I will be able to tell you my needs when asked through:	Introduce yourself to me and explain the purpose of your visit upon each contact. Call me by my name to capture my attention. Encourage me to verbalize/talk about my past interests (e.g., dolls, family). Encourage visits by my family/others. Place me near peers when I'm out of my room to give me an opportunity for mental and social stimulation. Talk to me about daily events or objects in my surroundings, and provide reminders/reassurance as appropriate during all contact with me. Offer to discuss with me facility happenings, seasons, holidays, simple current events, and familiar people. Provide me with social visits for connection with others throughout the day. Include me in sensory stimulation, Hands Alive, and massage. Invite, encourage, and help me to attend programs right before they start; target: music (polka, country, old-time, Lawrence Welk), special programs, church, rosary, Sunshine Group, and recreational games. Help me to pursue leisure interests by turning on the TV to talk shows, old movies, old programs, or Lawrence Welk; give me women's magazines to look at. Provide me with verbal and visual cues and direct physical guidance; use task segmentation and simple, clear directions for tasks within my abilities. Ask me for responses that I can provide. Emphasize my abilities and accomplishments. Redirect me to the task or activity at hand to my tolerance level, and provide tasks to help maintain my attention. When you hear me saying, "Hey, hey," stop and ask me what I need and provide reassurance that my needs will be met; often I just need a little TLC.	Discipline: All All All All All All All All All All All All All All	Date of review:

Dementia Program ACTIVITY CARE PLAN			Resident Name:	Room:	Medical Record #:	
Date written:	#5	My mood is variable and my responsiveness varies with my mood. I often sit with my eyes closed, but will open them when you prompt me to. I have a limited attention span and limited ability to focus. I am unable to follow most commands r/t my cognitive and physical impairment. I have periods of restlessness and agitation, and repetitive body motions/movement. I enjoy the multisensory room for its calming/soothing environment. I especially enjoy optical/visual and soothing stimuli. I do benefit from the environmental stimulation and variety in setting that some groups can provide.	I will spend time in social areas, especially the multisensory room, daily for social contact and environmental stimulation through: I will have comfort, decreased repetitive, spastic body movements, social connection with others, meaningful stimulation, and a variety of sensorial experiences each day through: I will utilize rocking w/c for comfort and relaxation through: I will have an improved attention span of 10 – 15 minutes within engaging small-group dementia-specific programming through:	Introduce yourself to me and explain your purpose upon each contact. Call me by my name to capture my attention. Encourage me to verbalize/talk about my past interests (e.g., my daughter Carol). Encourage visits by my family/others. Place me near peers when I'm out of my room to give me an opportunity for mental and social stimulation. Talk to me about daily events or objects in my surroundings, and provide reminders/reassurance as appropriate during all contacts. Offer to discuss with me facility happenings, seasons, holidays, simple current events, and familiar people. Provide me with social visits for connection with others throughout the day. Include me in sensory stimulation (especially visual/optical), Hands Alive, massage, outdoor walks (weather permitting), reading to me (short stories), softly brushing my hair, applying lotion, gentle hand massage or shoulder massage, and other soothing activities. Include me in programs of interest that offer a variety in setting; target: music (old-time, country, polka), special programs, church, small-group dementia-specific programs, and multisensory room programs. Provide me with simple, direct verbal and visual cues and direct physical guidance as needed to engage me in each activity. Provide reassurance as needed and assure my comfort level; if I look restless, look for signs of some physical need.	Discipline: All All All All All All All All All All All	Date of review:

Dementia Program ACTIVITY CARE PLAN				Resident Name: Room:	Medical Record #:	
				Use touch, activity equipment, and props to directly engage me in the activity.	All	
				Position in rocking w/c for periods of comfort and relaxation.	All	
				Redirect me to the activity/task to my tolerance by calling my name to capture my attention, gently touching me, and/or physically demonstrating actions.	All	
				Prompt me to open my eyes when I am holding them shut to increase my awareness of my environment.	All	

Short-Term Stay ACTIVITY CARE PLAN		Resident Name:		Room:		Medical Record #:
Date written:	#6	I expect to have a short-term stay at this facility for rehab. I had two previous short-term rehab stays here, so I am very familiar and comfortable with the facility and staff. I prefer independent activity, but would enjoy having one-to-one visits with the activities staff and may attend some groups. I am very social in nature and outgoing. I am able to self-structure my own day and I have many interests. I have a very supportive family and friends who visit daily.	I will participate in preferred independent leisure pursuits of interest—TV, reading, socializing/ reminiscing, and radio—during my stay through: I will interact with others on a daily basis and look forward to staff visits during my stay through:	Review the activities calendar with me to identify areas of interest. Introduce me to peers with similar interests and abilities, especially those who are also here for therapy. Stop in to see me to ensure that I am still content with my independent social and recreational contacts. Encourage independent leisure pursuits of interest; target: TV (golf, baseball, game shows, movies, and "Judge" shows), reading newspapers and women's magazines (Ladies Home Journal, Good Housekeeping, Women's Day, etc.), socializing with visitors, walking outdoors (weather permitting), reminiscing about my doll and bear collections and Tiger Woods paraphernalia, and listening to the radio. Inform me of groups of potential interest; target: music (polka), bingo, special programs, and socials. Have the volunteer library cart stop by my room so that I may check out magazines. I would love to have the activities director (who makes dolls) stop by and share her love of doll collecting with me and bring in some of her dolls for me to see.	Discipline: All All All All All All All	Date of review:

Long-Term Stay ACTIVITY CARE PLAN			Resident Name:	Room:	Medical Record #:
Date written:	#7	I am able to self-structure my own day and I am social in nature. I have peer friends I enjoy spending time with daily. I keep myself occupied with independent, low-energy-level activities. I have frequent family visits and my family takes me out a lot, especially on weekends, which I really look forward to. I often choose to do word searches, play cards, make crafts, or watch TV instead of joining in groups that are offered and are of expressed interest. I need to alternate rest with activity r/t SOB and I need to keep my legs elevated r/t CHF. I have a varying health status and my activity pursuits are reflective of my health.	I will continue to participate in independent leisure pursuits of interest daily and will ask for any assistance I may need to be able to pursue them through: I will interact/play cards with others daily, including playing cards with peers/friends in the evening, through: I will continue to go on outings with family members as I am able through: I will take an active role within groups as defined by the activity and as I am able through:	Encourage me to pursue my leisure interests—for example, TV (old movies/programs, westerns, "Perry Mason," "Little House on the Prairie"), reading (books: romance, historical; magazines), word searches, crosswords, casino machine, family visits/outings, jewelry-making, and other independent crafts (I like to take whatever craft we do as a group and then continue with more independence in my room). Invite me to attend, remind me of, and help me get to programs of interest; target: music (karaoke, Roger Ellis, Elvis impersonators, country, piano; I played piano in the past but have forgotten how), recreational games, dartball, crafts, socials, outings, gambling, dining out, shopping, table games, and discussion groups. Ask me open-ended questions to promote conversation and an active role. Remind me to rest throughout the day to reduce SOB. Remind me to alternate rest with activity. Encourage me to keep my legs elevated. Encourage my relationship with peers/friends and daily evening card-playing. Honor my wishes for independent activity over groups as I so choose.	Discipline: All All All All All All All All	Date of review:

Dementia Program ACTIVITY CARE PLAN				Resident Name:	Room:	Medical Record #:	
Date written:	#8	I have a very supportive family. I am new here, but I did live at a CBRF prior to coming here. I have very poor eyesight and hearing. I wear bilateral hearing aids and use a magnifier on my TV. I have problems concentrating and am forgetful, so I need reminders. I "tell it like it is" and I don't "beat around the bush."	I will demonstrate a feeling of adjustment by attending and actively participating in group activities through: I will spend time out of my room and by the aviary daily, as I like to watch the birds, through: I will offer discussion, respond to direct questions or statements, and complete simple one- and two-step tasks during small group activities through:	Introduce yourself and explain your purpose upon each contact. Call me by my name to capture my attention. Encourage me to verbalize/talk about my past interests (e.g., family, traveling). Encourage visits by my family/others. Place me near peers when I'm out of my room to provide me with mental and social stimulation. Talk to me about daily events or objects in my surroundings, and provide reminders/reassurance as appropriate during all contact with me. Offer to discuss with me facility happenings, seasons, holidays, simple current events, and familiar people. Provide me with social visits for connection with others throughout the day. Visit with me about my feelings regarding moving here and how I'm adjusting. Help me share and express my concerns. Help me meet other individuals who have similar interests and abilities. Encourage my involvement and decision-making in each aspect of daily life. Ask for my input regarding my preferences for daily routines, things I like to do, and group involvement. Provide me with assistive devices to ensure my ability to participate in leisure pursuits (e.g., magnifier on TV, hearing aides in place, seat me near speaker, provide me with additional verbal cues, speak directly and clearly to me during the program, offer one-on-one communication to further clarify the program's directions).	Discipline: All All All All All All All All All All All All	Date of review:

Long-Term Stay **ACTIVITY CARE PLAN**					**Resident Name:**	**Room:**	**Medical Record #:**	
					Offer seating for optimal vision and hearing at activities.	All		
					Praise me for all efforts and participation.	All		
					Encourage my leisure pursuits—for example, TV ("anything good," game shows, talk shows), family visits, and time spent by aviary.	All		
					Invite, encourage, and help me as needed to attend programs of potential interest; target: music (polka, country music, some classical), special events, recreational games, church, singalongs, and outings (out to eat, bus rides). Include me in sensory stimulation, Hands Alive, and massage.	All		

Long-Term Stay ACTIVITY CARE PLAN			Resident Name:	Room:	Medical Record #:	
Date written:	#9	I spend much of my day with my husband, who structures our time together with things we both enjoy. I prefer independent activity and time spent with my husband. I have minimal interests outside that.	I will continue to pursue leisure interests along with my husband on a daily basis through: I will continue to interact with others daily on a one-on-one basis through: I will welcome one-on-one activity visits evidenced by verbalizations and smiles through: I will continue to "check out" groups of interests with my husband through:	Review upcoming events with me and my husband to identify areas of interest and to keep me informed of what is going on in the facility. Include me in one-on-one activity visits for socialization and reminiscence. Encourage independent leisure pursuits of interest; target: TV (news, game shows), sitting outdoors (weather permitting), family visits, weekend trivia, and spending time out in activity areas observing what's going on. Invite and encourage both me and my husband to take part in groups of interest; target: special programs, music (country, old-time, big band, polka), church, and bingo. Greet us and make us feel welcome and included in groups we check out together. Ask open-ended question to promote conversation and an active role.	Discipline: All All All All All All	Date of review:

Long-Term Stay ACTIVITY CARE PLAN		Resident Name:	Room:	Medical Record #:	
Date written:	#10	I am social in nature, am willing to participate in activities as I am able, am able to self-structure my own day, and have leadership tendencies. I have had an exacerbation of my COPD and I get anxious at times r/t feeling as though I cannot catch my breath and large groups intensify this feeling. I become extremely SOB with exertion; I am SOB even at rest at times. I need to alternate rest with activity. I need materials for Red Hat Society pictures/ supplies to successfully assist the activities staff in maintaining a scrapbook.	I will continue to self-structure my day with low-energy-level activities of interest through: I will alternate rest with activity and will recognize my physical limitations to manage my SOB to the best of my ability through: I will take an active role as I am able by socializing with others, completing tasks within my abilities, and joining in topics of discussion with each activity through: I will participate in my preferred activity interest of helping others by maintaining a Red Hat scrapbook and assisting with mailings as I am able through:	Encourage me to continue to pursue low-energy–level, in-room activities of interest—for example, handheld games, TV (golf, game shows, "The Price is Right," soaps, evening programs, talk shows), reading (newspapers, magazines), socializing, family visits, outings (if up to it), weekend trivia, the casino machine, and solitaire. Invite, encourage as my health permits and I feel able, and help me to attend groups of interest; target: music (polka, country, old-time), special programs, socials, parties, bingo, recreational games, the resident council, the food committee, dartball, crafts, cooking club, church, rosary, volunteer tasks such as mailings, and outings as I am able (gambling, dining out, shopping). Provide me with Red Hat Society pictures and supplies to enable me to independently work on the scrapbooking activity, especially on weekends or when I feel unable to leave my room. Offer me one-on-one visits to provide needed independent materials for volunteer endeavors and to discuss my experiences and preferences. Encourage me to alternate rest with activity.	Discipline: All All All All All	Date of review:

Long-Term Stay ACTIVITY CARE PLAN			Resident Name:	Room:	Medical Record #:	
Date written:	#11	I have aphasia from my CVA. I am able to say one or two words in response. I am aware of and understand my surroundings. I do need time to respond. I have a supportive family, which is very important to me. I presently need assistance in structuring my day, but I prefer independent activity and time spent with my family. I may need adaptive devices to have successful experiences during activity programs r/t my CVA, right paresis, and poor eyesight.	I will participate in independent leisure pursuits of interest with staff/ family members set up through: I will interact with others on a daily basis and spend time out of my room daily for social opportunities through: I will complete simple tasks and verbally respond to simple questions/statements during each activity through: I will take part in the weekly recreational game by tossing/aiming for the target with school students' assistance through:	Encourage and assist me in participating in independent leisure pursuits of interest—for example, TV (channels 7, 9, and 20, public broadcasting, "Judge" shows, "Regis," sports), reading to me (short stories, magazine articles), helping me do a crossword by reading the clues and telling me the spaces and any letters already known, and reminiscing. Invite, encourage, and help me to attend programs of potential interest; target: music (waltz, polka; I used to love to dance), special programs, church, and recreational games. Cue me to look to my right side (weak side), and teach me ways to compensate. Place items in my left field of vision (e.g., targets for recreational games). Focus on my accomplishments during activity programs and praise my efforts. Provide verbal and visual cues and direct physical guidance for tasks within my abilities. Modify/simplify tasks (e.g., bring target closer and to my left side for recreational games). Make sure I have my glasses on for activities.	Discipline: All All All All All All	Date of review:

Dementia Program ACTIVITY CARE PLAN				Resident Name:	Room:	Medical Record #:	
Date written:	#12	I yell out at times and can be disruptive to groups. When asked why I yell, I usually do not even know that I am yelling. I love one-on-one attention, holding hands, physical contact so that I know someone is present, hand massages and shoulder massages, having short stories read to me, and conversations about simple topics. I like background country music playing on my radio when I am alone in my room. I have extremely poor eyesight and am very HOH. I often sit with my eyes shut.	I will respond to the best of my ability by opening my eyes when prompted, responding verbally to simple direct questions or statements, and squeezing/holding your hand during each activity/intervention through: I will spend time out of my room daily for social connections through: I will spend time in the multisensory room daily, with a focus on soothing, calming activities (e.g., relaxing music, bubble wall, waterfall curtain, aromatherapy, and water fountain) through:	Listen to, observe, and respond to my needs. Provide an unhurried pace. Sit with me at groups to provide an increased comfort level and human contact (hold my hand). Remove me from groups only if necessary to maintain a positive atmosphere and experience for all. Praise all of my positive social interactions. Include me in activities that I find comfortable and yet stimulating; target: massages, softly brushing my hair, touch, tactile and auditory stimulation (I like bird sounds, so turn those on in the multisensory room), country or relaxing CDs, reminiscing about my family, reading to me, and attending multisensory room programs. When I'm up, take me to be around other people so that I have frequent one-on-one staff contact. I like "The Golden Girls," the country music station, and old movies/programs on TV. Make sure the volume is at a level I can hear. Include me in sensory stimulation and Hands Alive. Include me in country music programs, special programs, and small-group dementia-specific programs that target reminiscence skills and social skills. Speak in a louder tone with enunciated speech and directly into my right ear. I hear best in one-on-one situations without background noise.	Discipline: All All All All All All All All All All All	Date of review:	

Dementia Program ACTIVITY CARE PLAN			Resident Name:	Room:	Medical Record #:	
Date written:	#13	I have limited concentration and decreased orientation to time and place. I like activities that promote a pleasant social environment. I often observe my surroundings and smile, as I am content to be among others. I enjoy having a variety of sensorial experiences each day. I especially enjoy holding comforting objects (stuffed animals) and items I can manipulate (PVC piping, as I was a plumber).	I will show you my pleasure and comfort by smiling and through my awareness of my environment by tracking movement (following actions by turning my head) through: I will have positive outcomes of increased responsiveness (verbal attempts) and physical movements (e.g., manipulating fiber optic bead curtain during multisensory room programs) through:	Introduce yourself and explain your purpose upon each contact.	Discipline: All	Date of review:
				Call me by my name to capture my attention.	All	
				Encourage me to verbalize/talk about my past interests (e.g., family, traveling, my work as a plumber).	All	
				Encourage visits by my family/others. Place me near peers when I'm out of my room to give me an opportunity for mental stimulation.	All	
				Talk to me about daily events or objects in my surroundings, and provide reminders/reassurance as appropriate during all contacts.	All	
				Offer to discuss with me facility happenings, seasons, holidays, simple current events, and familiar people.	All	
				Provide me with social visits for connection with others throughout the day.	All	
				Invite, encourage, and help me to attend programs of interest; target: music (country, polka, old-time), special programs, socials, church, and rosary.	All	
				Include me in sensory stimulation, massage, Hands Alive, and outdoor walks (weather permitting).	All	
				Set me up with manipulatives or give me soft objects (stuffed animals) I can hold for comfort, especially PVC piping/plumbing gadgets and other objects that can be turned. Take me by the aviary, as I enjoy watching the birds.	All	
				Ask me for responses you have confidence I can provide.	All	
				Provide me with verbal and visual cues and direct physical guidance.	All	

Dementia Program ACTIVITY CARE PLAN				Resident Name:	Room:	Medical Record #:	
				Simplify tasks for me and reduce environmental stimulation; give me extra time to respond.	All		
				Emphasize my abilities and accomplishments.	All		
				Prompt me for simple verbal responses of yes/no.	All		
				Include me in the multisensory room and in small-group dementia-specific programs; target manipulatives—things to handle and explore, and to see, to actively engage me in successful experiences.	All		

Dementia Program ACTIVITY CARE PLAN			Resident Name:	Room:	Medical Record #:	
Date written:	#14	I have periods of weepiness and varying receptiveness, moods, and levels of participation and become anxious at times. During those times I just want to be left alone in a calm environment. Other times I can be very social, enjoy being around others (actually preferring it to being alone), and am willing to take part in activities. You will need to gauge my mood upon approach.	I will have positive outcomes of decreased anxiousness/agitation/weepiness with use of the multisensory room (e.g., fiber optic bead curtain, bubble wall, water fountain, soothing music/nature sounds) through: I will complete a simple task, respond to simple questions with one or two words, or offer simple conversation on topics of discussion during small group programs through: I spend time in different social areas (multisensory room, activity areas, my own room alone) that match my current mood state and desires through:	Maintain my personal space until you gauge my present mood. Approach me slowly and from the front, using a calm and steady voice. Gently and firmly redirect me to an alternative activity or topic of conversation to reduce my anxiousness/agitation. Check to see whether I have an unmet physiological need. Offer me a quieter setting with soft music and slightly dimmed lighting as a sensory/environmental change. Include me in the multisensory room, which offers soothing activities and small-group dementia-specific programming that targets cognitive skills, reminiscence skills, and object identification; include me in the evening dementia program, as this calms me and helps me to have a good night. Ask me simple, direct questions related to the activity/topic at hand. Provide me with verbal and visual cues and direct physical guidance to engage me in each activity if I am open to it. Reminisce with me about pleasant life events (e.g., my daughter and husband). Offer me cookies to distract me from unpleasant thoughts. I do love my cookies! Provide me with needed reassurance; respond to my feelings and needs.	Discipline: All All All All All All All All	Date of review:

Dementia Program ACTIVITY CARE PLAN				Resident Name:	Room:	Medical Record #:	
Date written:	#15	I am nonverbal. I have minimal responses to activity interventions; I flinch to environmental sounds (loud or disturbing); I respond to my name and touch by opening my eyes; I smile, frown, raise my eyebrows, and blink my eyes in response to stimuli. I have very expressive facial expressions.

I like the visual stimulation provided by the multisensory room (e.g., fiber optic bead curtain, light projector, other items that light up and have motion). | I will observe my surroundings by following movement with my eyes through:

I will open my eyes, smile, or give another form of facial expression in response to contacts/stimuli through:

I will continue to spend time in various social areas for environmental stimulation opportunities through:

I will follow movement with my eyes (tracking) and turn my eyes toward sound during multisensory room interventions through: | Set me up with items that are stimulating and that increase my awareness of my environment; target: music CDs (hymns, country) and radio.

Position me when I'm in bed so that I can see my butterfly mobile in the window.

Set me up under the fiber optic waterfall, in front of the bubble wall, and turn other moving visual stimuli on in the multisensory room.

Give me verbal and visual prompts and simple statements to draw my attention to something, and observe me closely for responses to learn what I find pleasurable or what I dislike based on my facial expressions.

Position me in locations that enable me to have frequent one-on-one contact with others during activities and in social areas.

Provide hand-over-hand guidance to enable me to receive tactile stimulation.

Softly brush my hair, apply lotion or perfume (I will open my mouth when I smell pleasant aromas), or give me a gentle hand massage. Take me to different areas for a change of environment (e.g., aviary, activity room). Talk with me about my teaching and living in Alaska (I will usually raise my eyebrows when you talk about this).

Include me in sensory stimulation, Hands Alive, and massage. | Discipline: All

All

All

All

All

All

All

All | Date of review: |

Dementia Program ACTIVITY CARE PLAN				Resident Name:	Room:	Medical Record #:
Date written:	#16	I am social in nature and enjoy being around others and observing what is going on around me. I have severe cognitive decline with varying alertness and physical abilities r/t Parkinson's and dementia. I maintain large motor skills and the ability to mimic/mirror actions.	I will continue to "lead" an exercise sequence of upper-body large motor movements with activity staff assistance through: I will have positive outcomes of increased responsiveness and vocal attempts (respond to simple, direct questions or statements with one or two words) and will be able to mimic displayed actions/mirror actions during small-group dementia-specific programming and multisensory room programming through:	Invite, encourage, and help me to attend programs of interest; target: music (old-time, polka, country, jazz, and classical are my favorites), special programs, rosary, church, recreational games, trivia (I can still remember long-term, ingrained trivia), Sunshine Group, Five Alive, socials, outings (bus rides, city band concerts in the park to meet my wife there; my wife and I went every week our entire married life), and exercise (I have always been athletic, liked hiking and camping, and was a big outdoorsman). I have great pride in having been in the Navy, and my eyes light up and I smile broadly when you ask me about that part of my life. I will reminisce about it with you readily. Set me up with leisure pursuits of interest (e.g., the jazz/classical CD collection in my room; videos; westerns; also, I like to watch documentaries on TV). Take me by the aviary and other social areas, as I enjoy sitting and watching what is going on around me. Provide me with verbal and visual prompts so that I can help the staff "lead" exercises and to engage me in all activities as well as promote an active role. Modify interventions (more or less assistance/cueing) to fit my present alertness level and degree of physical abilities.	Discipline: All All All All All All	Date of review:

Long-Term Stay ACTIVITY CARE PLAN		Resident Name:		Room:	Medical Record #:	
Date written:	#17	I am very social in nature and enjoy interacting with others. I am able to self-structure my own day with independent activity, but I need reminders of groups of interest as I am forgetful. I am willing to participate in activities and I enjoy them. I do like to talk—a lot—and sometimes others may get a little annoyed with me. I am used to having things done the way I like them	I will continue to self-structure my own day through: I will continue to interact with others daily and have positive social experiences through: I will complete tasks as defined by the activity, offer discussion on topics, and socialize with others during each activity through:	Invite, encourage, and help me to attend programs of interest; target: music (polka, especially Chet and Gang as they are my favorite and I have a relative that plays in that band; waltz, country, and old-time), special programs, socials, church, rosary, bingo, discussion groups, dining out, theater, table games, and recreational games. Encourage leisure pursuits of interest—for example, TV (evening news only), reading (newspaper; I go to the office numerous times to get it until it comes, as I so look forward to this, and consequently have developed a friendship with the receptionist and we socialize daily), mail (I so look forward to receiving mail from my family and women's magazines from the library cart), going for "coffee breaks" throughout the day (I love my coffee), socializing with others I meet in social areas, crossword puzzles, and outdoor walks (weather permitting). Encourage my close relationship with my roommate. Remind me to let others have their time to express themselves during groups and interactions. Remind me to be more patient and understanding in my expectations.	Discipline: All All All All All	Date of review:

Long-Term Stay ACTIVITY CARE PLAN		Resident Name:		Room:	Medical Record #:	
Date written:	#18	I need to continue in my life-long established religious volunteer role here and in community connections with organizations for which I belong (e.g., Right to Life, homelessness advocate). I continue to identify strongly to past roles. I feel a strong sense of responsibility to my roles and take them all very seriously. I am able to self-structure my day and take on leadership roles with the nursing home and the community.	I will continue to self-structure my own day through: I will continue with my volunteer roles to the degree I am able through: I will attend, play organ for, lead the rosary, and participate in organizing Catholic church services, which have always been of significant importance to me, through: I will continue with my community connections via cell phone, open letters to the Journal, and writing letters to organizations through:	Remind me of programs of interest; target: Red Hat Society, rosary, church, bingo, recreational games, socials, resident council, food committee, stamps, chimes, music (hymns, polka, country, old-time, singalongs), special programs, trivia, and discussion groups. Encourage my leisure pursuits of interest—for example, TV (news, religious), reading (newspapers, books: biographies, romance, history; magazines: religious, reminiscence, country), crossword puzzles, outdoor walks (weather permitting), word searches, weekend trivia, solitaire, phone contacts, family visits, writing letters, and mail from organizations to which I belong. Praise me for my accomplishments and leadership roles. Encourage my volunteer roles: chapel services, leading rosary, community organization involvement, resident council, food committee, nursing home finance committee meetings, and leading the Saturday morning reading group.	Discipline: All All All All	Date of review:

Dementia Program ACTIVITY CARE PLAN				Resident Name:	Room:	Medical Record #:	
Date written:	#19	I do best in small groups with individualized attention r/t my short attention span, impaired cognition, poor eyesight, and virtually nonexistent hearing. (I do not use hearing devices, as they are ineffective.) I enjoy being around others, even though I do not socialize because of my impairments. I enjoy being by the activities leader during small groups, holding hands, and having the presence and physical contact. I feel comfortable with the staff members with whom I have developed a connection.	I will display my pleasure with participation by smiling and relaxing during the activity through: I will observe my surroundings and activities through: I will engage in small-group dementia-specific programming by covering game cards with the staff pointing out to me what to do, and mimicking/mirroring actions of the leader, through:	Use enunciated speech and cueing to foster my understanding. Pair me up with my daughter (also a resident) at large groups; she can assist me with knowing what bingo number to cover and provide some security. Reassure and accentuate my accomplishments. Invite, encourage, and help me to attend programs of interest; target: bingo, socials, exercise, Sunshine Group, recreational games, multisensory room programs (visual lights and motion), and small-group dementia-specific programming. Help me set up leisure interests—for example, family visits/daughter visits, DVDs of old programs, movies with children or animals, outdoor walks (weather permitting), and spending time in the multisensory room. Provide me with verbal cues (speak directly in my ear or in my line of vision as I can sometimes figure out what you are saying) and visual cues/gestures to aid in my understanding. Provide direct physical guidance to promote a physically engaged role. Sit with me at groups to help me to gain the most from the group setting and a social connection and to provide an element of security. I like to hold hands and to give hugs to those with whom I feel comfortable.	Discipline: All All All All All All All All	Date of review:

Long-Term Stay ACTIVITY CARE PLAN		Resident Name:		Room:	Medical Record #:	
Date written:	#20	I have many friends and family who are very supportive. I am able to self-structure my own day with activities of interest, which are primarily independent in nature as I am younger than most people here. I have MS and am a quadriplegic, so I have decreased strength and endurance. I use adaptive devices to maintain as much independence as possible, and this remains very important to me. I use a mouthpiece, page turner, book holder, voice-activated computer, speaker phone, and special call cord that I activate by nodding my head, all of which enable my independence.	I will maintain my social contacts via phone, e-mail, and in-person visits daily through: I will continue to pursue leisure interests with staff setup and use of my adaptive devices through: I will socially participate in church, rosary, prayer groups, the Red Hat Society, and independent outings with family/friends weekly through:	Visit with me one-on-one for socialization and to determine any activity needs I may have. Invite, encourage, and help me to attend predetermined activity groups of interest; target: music (Gene Hersey, country/guitar players), some socials and special programs, Red Hat Society, theater, concerts in the park, picnics, out to eat, and shopping. Assist me with needs associated with leisure pursuits of putting in videos/DVDs, watching TV (turning to talk shows, movies), using the phone (have it near me with my mouthpiece), and using the computer (e-mail, Internet, letter writing, poetry writing, reading the newspaper online; set me up at my desk). Send me the activities schedule via e-mail and point out programs of potential interest. Encourage me to focus on my accomplishments by providing sincere praise. Encourage and support weekly outings with use of the community van. (I participate in fewer outings in extreme cold or hot weather as that is more taxing on me r/t my MS.)	Discipline: All All All All All All	Date of review:

Chapter 3

Holidays, Birthdays, Special Events, and Themed Activities

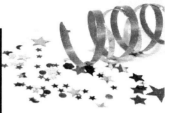

Celebrations are a big part of our lives. They help define who we are. They make us feel special, loved, needed, and cared for. Celebrations are opportunities for socialization and recognition, which are psychological needs we have throughout our lives. They afford us the opportunity to gather together as a larger community. They provide us with opportunities for reminiscence and for building/maintaining friendships and connections with others.

Social opportunities play a role in maintaining wellness. The social dimension of wellness encourages contributing to one's environment and community. It emphasizes the interdependence between others and nature, being more aware of society and the impact you have on the environment, preserving the beauty and balance of nature, and discovering the power to make willful choices to enhance personal relationships, establish important friendships, and build a better living space and community.

A person with social wellness:

- Has and maintains satisfying relationships

- Practices good communication skills

- Cultivates a support network of caring friends and family members

- Enjoys the friendship of people with diverse backgrounds and ethnic origins

- Participates in service projects and demonstrates concern for others

- Can appreciate lifestyles and opinions which may be different from his or her own

- Volunteers in the community

- Becomes involved in organizations/groups/clubs

Share some or all of the following activities with the residents in your community. They will help you preserve your residents' social wellness, sense of self, importance, and social skills.

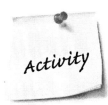

Activity | '50s Day

Target audience: Residents who enjoy social opportunities, based on resident interests and needs, especially residents who enjoyed the 1950s

Objectives/outcomes:

- Promotes social interaction between peers and the staff, mental stimulation, and recreation

- Provides for companionship, refreshments, and conversation

- Provides a learning opportunity

- Provides an opportunity for reminiscence, which promotes mental stimulation, long-term memory skills, and cognitive/thinking skills

- Trivia/discussion groups: promote mental stimulation, long-term memory skills, and cognitive/thinking skills

Recommended group size: Small or large (varies based on activity)

Suggested time frame: 30 – 60 minutes for each activity

Special needs/ability level (physical/cognitive skills needed): Primarily residents with moderate to high cognitive functioning. Ability to follow directions, complete tasks, respond verbally, and interact on some level.

Activity outline:

- Have the Dietary Department plan a "carhop" luncheon (hamburgers, French fries, soda, and ice cream sundaes). Have the staff dress as carhops and serve the residents their meals. Promote conversations with open-ended questions and encourage peer conversations. Play background 1950s music to set the mood (in all dining areas), and to develop a pleasant and appropriate atmosphere.

- Have an afternoon or early evening sock hop. "Spin" some 1950s music yourself or secure a deejay if that is within your budget. Secure a school group or other volunteers to come and help residents to "jive" to the music. Have the staff/volunteers do the limbo while residents observe. Serve cherry soda or soda floats as refreshments.

- Have a root beer float social. Make the root beer floats in the residents' presence and serve them right away before they become soupy. Play background 1950s music.

- Have a hula hoop contest with the staff as contestants and residents as spectators (this will elicit laughter). Whoever keeps the hula hoop going the longest wins (you may need to set a time frame if you have staff member[s] who seem like they will never tire).

- Have a 1950s trivia contest. Get your information from books or off the Internet.

- Have a 1950s fad discussion group. Get your information from books or off the Internet.

For each activity, always welcome everyone to the group and always close the activity with a "Goodbye" and "See you next time." Praise and thank everyone for participating.

Variations/adaptations/modifications: Some of the activities may be offered one-on-one with residents who are unwilling or unable to participate in a group. You will need to simplify tasks, make adaptations (certain residents may need closer targets, or verbal and visual cues), and offer more assistance to those residents with diminished abilities (e.g., they may be able to perform tasks with direct hand-over-hand guidance). Some activities can include low-functioning residents when adaptations/modifications are made. You can use the format discussed here for a 1960s, '70s, '80s, or '90s day; just change the activities to go with the decade. You can also "Celebrate the Decades" activity and hold a 1920s, '30s, '40s, '50s, '60s, '70s, '80s, and '90s day each day.

Helpful hints/notes: Decorate the dining and activity areas in a 1950s theme. Encourage residents and the staff to dress in 1950s attire for the day. Observe all infection-control guidelines and individual resident dietary needs/restrictions when serving food and beverages. Much of the setup for the events can be done prior to gathering the residents so that you are ready to begin once residents have gathered. Assemble all needed equipment and supplies prior to the start of each activity. Save all the information you've gathered for this event, laminate it or put it in plastic sleeves, and place it in a binder or folder labeled "1950s Day," and you now have an annual event already planned for years to come.

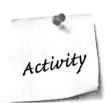

Activity | Annual King and Queen of Hearts Dance

Target audience: All residents, family members, and staff members who enjoy music and social events, based on resident needs and interests

Objectives/outcomes:

- To provide a festive Valentine's Day dance/party setting for all and a special time of socializing, and bring the community/junior high school students together with your residents

- Is great PR for your Activities Department/facility

- Provides for companionship, recognition, refreshments, and conversation

Recommended group size: Large; open to all residents, family members, and the community

Suggested time frame: Two hours

Activity outline:

- Materials and equipment: You will need a space that is large enough to accommodate the event; chairs; camera/film; music/entertainment that people can dance to; refreshments coordinated between the Dietary and Activities departments; napkins and cups; king and queen crowns and scepters; and corsages and boutonnières.

- Decorations and centerpieces: Valentine's Day-themed balloons and other Valentine's Day decorations to set the mood; a trellis or archway decorated in a Valentine's Day theme.

- Preparation, planning, and participation: Plan to hold the event on the weekend closest to Valentine's Day (this allows residents' family members to attend). Planning this activity is similar to planning a prom.

  - You will need to find a group to take this on, as most Activities departments don't have enough staff members to carry out the event; suggest a junior high or high school club. Such a club should provide you with students who can attend the event.

The school may also pay for the band that day if you request it.

– The Dietary Department should provide punch and cookies.

– About a month prior to the event, the teachers/chaperones and you should select the date of the event. You should plan to hold the event from 2 p.m. to 4 p.m. on the Saturday or Sunday closest to Valentine's Day.

– Arrange for a polka band or other band per your residents' preference.

– Two to three weeks prior to the event, ask the unit staff to select one female resident and one male resident to serve on the court. Have the court consist of one couple from each unit.

– Type up ballots and put them in staff members' paychecks so that the entire nursing home staff can vote for a King of Hearts and a Queen of Hearts. Every resident on the ballot is on the court. The names of the King and Queen of Hearts are kept secret until you announce them on the day of the event, during the coronation.

– The day of the event, each lady of the court receives a pink carnation corsage and each male of the court receives a red carnation boutonnière. It is nice to order real flowers from a florist and have them delivered. They may give you a discount, as they become familiar with the event.

– Hold the coronation at 2:30 p.m. and announce the king and queen. Present the winners with a king's crown and queen's tiara, as well as a scepter for each. This can be costly, but you can reuse them from year to year. Buy good-quality accessories (not cardboard, which doesn't last).

– Make every resident on the court feel special for the day, not just the king and queen. Have a dance for just the court, and pair students with residents to escort them around the dance floor. The students should dance with all residents who are willing, even those in wheelchairs. Utilize the Valentine's Day trellis for this event; the residents and students can parade/dance through it throughout the afternoon.

– Families should be encouraged to attend this event.

– The staff should dress residents in their "Sunday best" (red and pink colors are promoted) for this event.

– Invite the local paper to write a story and/or take a picture.

Helpful hints/notes: Decorate the activity area in a Valentine's Day theme. Observe all infection-control guidelines and individual resident dictary needs/restrictions when serving food and beverages. You must know of any food allergies your residents may have. Much of the setup for the event can be done prior to gathering residents so that you are ready to begin once residents have gathered. Assemble all needed equipment and supplies prior to the start of the activity. Save all information gathered for this event, laminate it or put it in plastic sleeves, and place it in a binder or folder labeled "Annual King and Queen of Hearts Valentine's Day Dance," and you now have an annual event already planned for years to come.

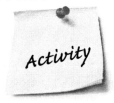

Annual Sweetheart Dinner

Target audience: All married residents with living spouses. This event is open only to married residents. Include short-term Medicare residents in this event, as they go back out in the community and talk about how special they felt.

Objectives/outcomes:

- To provide a special Valentine's Day event and time of socializing for married residents and their spouses

- Is great PR for your Activities Department/facility

- Provides for companionship/maintenance of lifelong relationships, recognition, a shared meal, and conversation

- Promotes feelings of love/romance, importance, and acceptance

- Promotes reminiscence

Recommended group size: Will depend on how many married residents currently reside in your facility

Suggested time frame: One to two hours

Special needs/ability level (physical/cognitive skills needed): Make modifications as needed to allow all married residents the opportunity to take part, with the exception of residents who would be NPO (nothing by mouth).

Activity outline:

- This event requires significant planning and coordination, especially because the census changes so rapidly for nursing homes.

- Aim to hold this event on Valentine's Day, unless February 14 falls on a weekend, in which case hold the event the Friday before or Monday after Valentine's Day.

- About a month prior to the event, go through the resident roster and identify those residents who have a spouse. Do this up to the day of the event; so, if a resident moves in the day before the event and has a spouse, include them both in the event if possible. This means you have to plan for some extra "couples" when doing your initial planning.

- Design beautiful invitations (you can subscribe to AmericanGreetings.com as one option for creating invites). Make sure you include the event name, date, time, and location and note that it is exclusively for married residents and spouses. There is a good chance that spouses may ask whether their children can be included. This request cannot be accommodated, usually for two reasons. First, you wouldn't have the space to accommodate everyone. And second, your goal is to make this a romantic event for married residents and their spouses, and if you allow their children to come, you cannot rightly bar single residents from the event, as most have children they could invite as their sweethearts and the facility's cost for the meal for that many attendees would be prohibitive. Send an invitation to each couple two weeks before the event. Have them RSVP a week prior to the event so that you can provide a food count to the Dietary Department (again allowing for extra, due to the potential for new admits to your facility).

- The Dietary Department should plan a special meal at no charge to the couples. You can serve that same meal to the other residents that day, as they should have a special meal as well.

- Arrange to have a barbershop quartet come in during the meal to deliver singing telegrams to your guests, and have them present a Valentine's Day card as well as a single, long-stemmed red rose to each couple. The cost for this is worth the residents'/ spouses' positive experience and the PR you will get from this event.

- Plan for your guests to arrive at least 30 minutes prior to serving the meal. As the guests arrive, place them under a trellis archway that is decorated for Valentine's Day and take their "Sweetheart Picture." Take two pictures with a Polaroid camera and two with a digital camera. Give the couple one of the Polaroid photos to keep that day. Then escort the couples to their seats.

- Prior to the event, you should make place cards for assigned seating (decorated for Valentine's Day, of course), as well as place settings. Consider each couple and with whom you think they will strike up conversations and have similar backgrounds/ interests. Many of your residents/spouses know other residents/spouses.

- Set the tables as you might find them in a high-end restaurant, with tablecloths and real floral arrangements. (You can use candles, but you cannot light them; use battery-powered candles instead.)

- The Activities Department and management should serve as hosts/hostesses as well as the wait staff. Have appropriate staff members available to assist any residents who need dining assistance. Serve the meal restaurant style, not on trays.

Variations/adaptations/modifications: Sometimes family members may want to take part in the meal, but not in a group situation. You can accommodate this request by setting up family members for the special meal in the residents' rooms. You can bring them their rose and Valentine's Day card; however, they would miss out on the entertainment.

Helpful hints/notes: Decorate the activity area in a Valentine's Day theme. Have floral centerpieces on all the tables. Observe all infection-control guidelines and individual resident dietary needs/restrictions when serving food and beverages. You must know of any food allergies your residents and their guests may have. Much of the setup for the event can be done prior to gathering the residents so that you are ready to begin once residents arrive. Assemble all needed equipment and supplies prior to the start of the activity. Save all information gathered for this event, laminate it or put it in plastic sleeves, and place it in a binder or folder labeled "Annual Sweetheart Dinner," and you now have an annual event already planned for years to come.

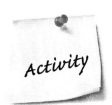

Activity

Back-to-School Week (August or September Event)

Target audience: Residents who enjoy social opportunities, based on their interests and needs, especially residents who were schoolteachers

Objectives/outcomes:

- Promotes social interaction between peers and the staff, mental stimulation, and recreation.

- Provides for companionship, refreshments, and conversation.

- Provides a learning opportunity.

- Provides an opportunity for reminiscence, which promotes mental stimulation, long-term memory skills, and cognitive/thinking skills.

- Trivia/discussion groups: promote mental stimulation, long-term memory skills, and cognitive/thinking skills.

- Recreational games and recess games: promote physical activity and engagement. Provide opportunities for physical exercise and for residents to enjoy friendly competition in a recreational setting. Benefits include maintaining and improving gross motor skills, maintaining and improving hand-eye coordination, and developing a sense of pride and self-esteem associated with friendly competition and team play.

Recommended group size: Small or large (varies based on activity)

Suggested time frame: 30 – 60 minutes for each activity

Special needs/ability level (physical/cognitive skills needed): Primarily residents with moderate to high cognitive functioning. Ability to follow directions, complete tasks, respond verbally, and interact on some level.

Activity outline:

- Reading, writing, and arithmetic discussion group or sensory group: This can be conducted as a small to medium-size group or one-on-one as a sensory program. Have a schoolbook bag (or backpack, though residents did not use those) filled with a ruler, pencil, pencil case, chalk, small "slate" board, crayons, watercolor paints, spelling list, penmanship paper, miniature globe, Dick and Jane book(s), books or articles on school days, song sheets for "Good Old School Days," and other school-related items. Have a discussion of school days—the differences between then and now (one-room school versus today's schools, walking versus taking the bus, discipline, etc.). Read stories out of books or articles and promote reminiscence (this activity can be led by the activities director, or residents can read aloud, as even residents with moderate cognitive impairments can still read simple stories). Practice some good penmanship and talk about the importance of this. Do some arithmetic on a large blackboard or have some sheets run off with addition, subtraction, multiplication, and division problems. Recite the alphabet. Recite the "Pledge of Allegiance" (have a flag for them to face, and have them put their hand over their heart), and discuss feelings among residents about the fact that schools no longer do this. Adapt what you do to the physical and cognitive functioning level of each participant.

- Recess fun: Play dodge ball with the staff in the center of the circle and residents kicking/rolling a large ball (such as those used for ball exercise classes). Use a parachute and have residents take turns moving it up and down, making waves, and so on. Have residents try their hand at jacks or marbles if they are able. They can at least touch/feel them and reminisce about the games they used to play during recess (hopscotch, jump rope; see what games they can remember).

- Spelling bee: Use a spelling bee book or come up with word lists of your own from the dictionary. Even residents with moderate cognitive loss can still spell. Give words according to individual resident abilities so that each resident is successful yet challenged by this activity. Make it a friendly competition.

- Geography bee: Utilize books, teaching resources, or the Internet for information. Display a large world map, state map, local map, and globe.

- History facts discussion group/trivia: Utilize books, teaching resources, or the Internet for information. Ask residents to name some important events in history and discuss them.

- Science facts discussion group/trivia: Utilize books, teaching resources, or the Internet for information. Find a simple science experiment that you can demonstrate.

- Have a weather forecaster come and talk about his or her work, various forms of weather, and how weather predictions are made.

- Schedule a "field trip" (though residents didn't take them, their children may have) to the local library, museum, TV station, fire station, or other place of interest to your residents that might be an area which school children would visit on a class trip.

- Have a school class visit and do an activity with the residents. Read stories aloud, play bingo, or play a recreational game (ring toss, horse shoes, bean bag toss, Frisbee toss, basketball, golf putting, etc.).

- Have a children's jump rope group come and demonstrate the skills of jumping rope.

- Schedule snack time, and serve milk and animal crackers.

For each activity, always welcome everyone to the group and always close the activity with a "Goodbye" and "See you next time." Praise and thank everyone for their participation.

Variations/adaptations/modifications: Some of the activities may be offered one-on-one with residents who may be unwilling or unable to participate in a group. You will need to simplify tasks, make adaptations (certain residents may need closer targets, or verbal and visual cues), and offer more assistance to some residents who have diminished abilities (they may be able to perform tasks with direct hand-over-hand guidance). Some activities can include low-functioning residents when adaptations/modifications are made.

Helpful hints/notes: Decorate the dining and activity areas in a "back-to-school" theme. Observe all infection-control guidelines and individual resident dietary needs/restrictions when serving food and beverages. Much of the setup for these events can be done prior to gathering residents so that you are ready to begin once the residents have gathered. Assemble all needed equipment and supplies prior to the start of each activity. Encourage a positive atmosphere for fair, fun recreational play and competition. Announce and congratulate winners and players. Watch for signs of residents becoming overly tired or too competitive. Save all the information you've gathered for this event, laminate it or put it in plastic sleeves, and place it in a binder or folder labeled "Back-to-School Week," and you now have an annual event already planned for years to come.

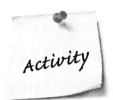
Activity

Beach/Hawaiian Day

Target audience: Residents who enjoy social opportunities, based on resident interests and needs

Objectives/outcomes:

- Promotes social interaction between peers and the staff, mental stimulation, and recreation

- Provides for companionship, refreshments, and conversation

- Provides a learning opportunity

- Surfin' safari beach volleyball, pineapple toss, and coconut bowling: provide opportunities for physical exercise and friendly competition in a recreational setting

- To maintain and improve fine and gross motor skills

- To maintain and improve hand-eye coordination

- To develop in residents a sense of pride and self-esteem associated with friendly competition and team play

Recommended group size: Small or large (varies based on activity)

Suggested time frame: 30 – 60 minutes for each activity

Special needs/ability level (physical/cognitive skills needed): Primarily residents with moderate to high cognitive functioning. Ability to follow directions, complete tasks, respond verbally, and interact on some level.

Activity outline:

- Surfin' safari beach volleyball: You will need a net (or something similar to define the two sides for the teams) and a beach ball (regular size). Place six to 10 residents on each side to represent each team (we use more residents than a regular volleyball game, as it's easier on residents physically and gets more residents actively involved at one time). The remaining residents can watch, and then can switch with those who were playing (if they are physically able) so that they can have a turn. If residents are able to serve, have them serve; otherwise, a staff member can toss the ball into the middle of the playing area and play can begin from there. Encourage residents to keep the beach ball volleying as long as possible. Keep score for the two teams. You may want to decide on a winning number before starting, as usually the residents will tire long before a score of 15 is reached, as in regular volleyball. (It really depends on the ability levels of your residents.) Whatever rules you decide, make sure you announce them prior to starting the game.

- Have the Dietary Department plan a beach/Hawaiian dinner for all residents. Promote conversations with open-ended questions and encourage peer conversations. Play beach-themed music in the background (e.g., the Beach Boys) or Hawaiian music to set the mood (in all of the dining areas) and to develop a pleasant and appropriate atmosphere.

- Have a Hawaiian luau. Play Hawaiian music, secure hula dancers or have staff members participate in a hula contest (have grass skirts on hand for the staff to wear while performing), and have residents vote on the best hula dancer. Serve frozen drinks (see the following bulleted item) or other traditional Hawaiian drinks. This activity is usually held with a large group.

- Have a frozen drink social some afternoon. You should be able to secure the mixes through your Dietary Department and their food vendor. Frozen-drink mixes come in strawberry and piña colada flavors and you can make them with or without alcohol. Be sure to make the drinks in the residents' presence and serve them immediately so that they are nice and frozen. Place chopped fresh pineapple and a strawberry on toothpicks and place one toothpick in each glass. Don't forget the little umbrellas, too! Play background beach or Hawaiian music or have a steel-guitar player come and entertain if available. Promote conversations with open-ended questions and encourage peer conversations. This is generally a large group activity, but you can hold this activity for small groups on individual units or in the form of a "Treat Cart" whereby you visit each resident in his or her room. Although this latter approach is good for residents who cannot or will not attend group activities, you will lose the socialization aspect doing it this way.

- Have a Hawaiian trivia contest. You can get the trivia for this contest from the Internet. You can conduct this activity in a small or large group, or one-on-one in each resident's room.

- Show a Hawaiian travel video/DVD (or a video/DVD of any beach destination). You can conduct this activity in a small or large group, or as an independent, in-room activity.

- Play ring the pineapple and coconut bowling. You will need to purchase several fresh pineapples and coconuts ahead of time. For ring the pineapple, place two whole fresh pineapples on the floor as the targets and give each resident a set of rings (we use rings from our ring toss game). Have them take turns tossing the rings, trying to ring the pineapple. Residents receive one point for each ring they make and half a point for a "leaner." Keep score; the person with the highest score wins the game. For coconut bowling, place three bowling pins (we use bowling pins from our bowling game, but have reduced the number as it's harder to bowl with coconuts) on the floor. Give each resident a coconut to roll at the pins. Play and score as you would for normal bowling (you may not want to play 10 frames, but decide on this ahead of time and announce all the rules before beginning the game). Residents can play this game on the floor (set the pins 8 feet away from the residents) or on an 8-foot tabletop, but note that it can be challenging to keep the coconuts on the table at times.

For each activity, always welcome everyone to the group and always close the activity with a "Goodbye" and "See you next time." Praise and thank everyone for their participation.

Variations/adaptations/modifications: Some of the activities may be offered one-on-one for residents who are unwilling or unable to participate in a group. You will need to simplify tasks, make adaptations (certain residents may need closer targets, or verbal and visual cues), and offer more assistance to those residents with diminished abilities (they may be able to perform tasks with direct hand-over-hand guidance). Some activities can include low-functioning residents when adaptations/modifications are made.

Helpful hints/notes: Decorate the dining and activity areas in a beach/Hawaiian theme. Encourage residents and staff members to dress in beach/Hawaiian attire for the day. Observe all infection-control guidelines and individual resident dietary needs/restrictions when serving food and beverages. You must know of any food allergies your residents may have. Much of the setup for these events can be done prior to gathering residents so that you are ready to begin once the residents have gathered. Assemble all needed equipment and supplies prior to the start of each activity. Encourage a positive atmosphere for fair, fun recreational play and competition. Announce and congratulate winners and players. Watch for signs of residents becoming overly tired or too competitive. Save all the information you've gathered for this event, laminate it or put it in plastic sleeves, and place it in a binder or folder labeled "Beach/ Hawaiian Day," and you now have an annual event already planned for years to come.

Activity   Birthday Party

Target audience: Residents who enjoy social opportunities and are celebrating a birthday, based on resident interests and needs

Objectives/outcomes:

- Promotes social interaction among peers, family members, and the staff

- Provides for companionship and conversation

- Promotes reminiscence

- Provides opportunities for recognition and builds self-esteem

Recommended group size: Varies

Suggested time frame: One hour

Special needs/ability level (physical/cognitive skills needed): All residents can participate on some level.

Activity outline:

- Plan a facility-wide birthday party in which birthday celebrants and others celebrate on a selected day each month. Schedule a band/musical entertainer of resident preference. Be sure to announce the name of each resident celebrating his or her birthday and the date of each resident's birthday, sing "Happy Birthday," and serve birthday cake and punch. Schedule this event routinely (e.g., the last Friday of the month at 2 p.m.).

- Hold a small birthday party or tea. Schedule it routinely (e.g., the third Tuesday of every month at 2 p.m.). Only residents who are actually celebrating a birthday that month are invited. Recognize each person's birthday; serve cake and punch or tea.

- Recognize individual birthdays on the day of each resident's birthday. Have a birthday poster listing names and dates of birthdays only (no years of birth). Give the celebrant a birthday cupcake during the noon meal, and have the staff present it as restaurants do: A group approaches the resident with the cupcake and they sing "Happy Birthday" to the celebrant. Give each celebrant a card and/or balloon on the morning of his or her birthday. This will make others aware and prompt them to wish the celebrant happy birthday throughout the day. You can easily make cards on a computer. Or you can routinely conduct a craft-stamping activity during which residents make birthday cards so that you will have a stock of cards on hand.

- Hold an on-unit/household birthday gathering on each celebrant's actual birthday. This works best in household settings where there are fewer residents and the atmosphere is more family-like, but it is not impossible to hold on larger units. Have this be a unit staff activity (not an Activities Department activity). This will promote other staff members to do group activities and free the activities staff to focus on other events/activities. Staff members should recognize the celebrant, serve birthday cake and punch, and present a small gift. Sometimes family members will sponsor this event in recognition of their loved one.

For each activity, always welcome everyone to the group and always close the activity with a "Goodbye" and "See you next time." Praise and thank everyone for their participation.

Variations/adaptations/modifications: Some activities can be done on a one-on-one basis for those who cannot or will not take part in group activities. Instead of music/entertainment for the facility-wide birthday party, play birthday bingo and have wrapped prizes that residents can select from. (Be sure to mark each item as being either for a man, for a woman, or generic. Prizes should be such that anyone could use them—for example, lotion, perfume, aftershave, jewelry, etc.). Ask church groups to sponsor the monthly birthday parties (i.e., provide refreshments, small gifts for the celebrants, and volunteers to assist at the event).

Helpful hints/notes: Decorate the activity area in a birthday theme. Much of the setup for the event can be done prior to gathering residents so that you are ready to begin once the residents have gathered. Observe all infection-control guidelines and individual resident dietary needs/restrictions when serving food and beverages. Assemble all needed equipment and supplies prior to the start of each activity.

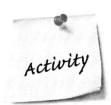

Activity

Camping Week (or Day)

Target audience: Residents who enjoy social opportunities, especially those who enjoyed camping activities and getting outdoors, based on resident interests and needs

Objectives/outcomes:

- Promotes social interaction among peers, family members, and the staff.

- Provides for companionship and conversation.

- Promotes reminiscence, mental stimulation, long-term memory skills, and cognitive/ thinking skills.

- Provides a learning opportunity.

- The sights, scents, sounds, and connection with nature promote positive memories and a connection to meaningful feelings.

- Exercise and recreational games: provide opportunities for physical exercise and to enjoy friendly competition in a recreational setting. Maintain and improve fine and gross motor skills and maintain and improve hand-eye coordination.

- To develop a sense of pride and self-esteem associated with friendly competition and team play.

- Crafts: allow residents to express their creative ideas. Promote residents' self-esteem through successful projects. Maintain and develop fine motor skills and hand-eye coordination. Provide residents with an opportunity for choice and preference in regard to the finished project.

Recommended group size: Small to large (varies based on activity)

Suggested time frame: 30 – 60 minutes for each activity

Special needs/ability level (physical/cognitive skills needed): Primarily residents with moderate to high cognitive functioning. Ability to follow directions, complete tasks, respond verbally, and interact on some level.

Activity outline:

- Attempt to conduct all activities outdoors if the weather cooperates; some activities can be held indoors, but the idea is to get residents out and experience the "camping" feeling. Some activities can be held off-campus at campgrounds/parks if you have that option and resident interests/abilities indicate it as such. Otherwise, make your campus grounds feel and look like a camp area. Borrow a tent, camping gear, fire pit, and other camping items from staff members to have set up for the week. Have tables and chairs set up in the same area for the week. Schedule enough volunteer help for each activity. Don't forget sunscreen, hats/visors, and sunglasses for outdoor activities, and encourage plenty of fluids.

- Every morning, schedule a short (10- or 15-minute) "wake-up" activity: an outdoor walk, or a stretching exercise. Enjoy the birds, nature, and so on. Consider it a pre-activity to your main morning event.

- After the "wake-up" activity, have a craft activity planned. For example, make pine-cone/peanut butter bird feeders and hang them from trees on campus; create leaf rubbings and place them between clear contact paper and in a frame; decorate base-ball caps and/or visors with fabric paint; make a group quilt with precut squares and fabric paint related to camping/outdoor activities; and/or tie-dye T-shirts or make "I Survived Camp Week at [your facility name]" T-shirts as a good activity for the end of the week.

- Every afternoon, schedule a camp recreational game: golf putting, horseshoes, bocce ball, beanbag toss, shuffle board, basketball, lawn jarts, and so on.

- On at least one evening, have a campfire, sing campfire songs (have a musician playing guitar stroll among the campers or play CDs of campfire songs), roast marshmallows, make s'mores (or other campfire recipes), eat popcorn, and drink lemonade. Encourage residents' family members to attend this event.

- Take residents on a fishing trip to a handicapped accessible spot one morning or afternoon.

- Have at least one cookout/grill-out during the week. Serve hot dogs, hamburgers, bratwurst, condiments, baked beans, potato salad, and cookies.

- Though residents would not be able to go horseback riding, you may be able to schedule someone to bring miniature horses to your facility so that residents can see, pet, and hear about them.

- Schedule a pontoon boat ride for your residents as a special outing during this week. Have your administrator captain the boat.

- Schedule a picnic at an area park that is part of a campground, and then have the residents sit by the lake. If they are able, have them take off their shoes, feel the grass under their feet, and dip their toes into the water or the warm sand.

For each activity, always welcome everyone to the group and always close the activity with a "Goodbye" and "See you next time." Praise and thank everyone for their participation.

Variations/adaptations/modifications: Some of the activities may be offered one-on-one with residents who are unwilling or unable to participate in a group. You will need to simplify tasks, make adaptations (certain residents may need closer targets, or verbal and visual cues), and offer more assistance to residents who have diminished abilities (they may be able to perform tasks with direct hand-over-hand guidance). Some activities can include low-functioning residents when adaptations/modifications are made.

Helpful hints/notes: If you are able to hold only a camping day from among the other activities on the list, you will not be able to hold all of the aforementioned events. Pick and choose the ones that would be of greatest interest to your residents. Observe all infection-control guidelines and individual resident dietary needs/restrictions when serving food and beverages. Much of the setup for these events can be done prior to gathering residents so that you are ready to begin once the residents have gathered. Assemble all needed equipment and supplies prior to the start of each activity. Encourage a positive atmosphere for fair, fun recreational play and competition. Save all the information you've gathered for this event, laminate it or put it in plastic sleeves, and place it in a binder or folder labeled "Camping Week," and you now have an annual event already planned for years to come.

Chinese New Year Theme Day

Target audience: Residents who enjoy social opportunities, and especially those with an ethnic background, based on resident interests and needs

Objectives/outcomes:

- Promotes social interaction between peers and staff, mental stimulation, and recreation

- Provides for companionship, refreshments, and conversation

- Provides a cultural and learning opportunity

- Craft and cooking class: Allows residents to express their creative ideas. Promotes residents' self-esteem through successful projects. Maintains and develops fine motor skills and hand-eye coordination. Provides residents with an opportunity for choice and preference in regard to the finished project.

Recommended group size: Small or large (varies based on activity)

Suggested time frame: 30 – 60 minutes for each activity

Special needs/ability level (physical/cognitive skills needed): Primarily residents with moderate to high cognitive functioning. Ability to follow directions, complete tasks, respond verbally, and interact on some level.

Activity outline:

- Morning activity: Offer an origami demonstration and/or have an origami craft session. You can purchase origami instructional books, borrow books from the library, or research the subject on the Internet ahead of time. The group size for this activity should be small—one staff member per resident. This also can be offered in residents' rooms. Play Chinese music in the background during this activity if it is not distracting.

- Luncheon activity: Have the Dietary Department prepare a Chinese dinner for all residents, order Chinese take-out from an authentic Chinese restaurant and have it delivered, or go out to eat to a Chinese restaurant. If the residents will be eating at the facility, play Chinese music to set the mood (in all of the dining areas) and to develop a pleasant and appropriate atmosphere. Promote conversations with open-ended questions and encourage peer conversations. You can offer a fun (and perhaps humorous) opportunity for residents by providing them with chopsticks as an alternative to silverware. This activity can be held for a small group (ordering take-out) or a large group when the Dietary Department prepares the food for all the residents and they dine in their regular dining areas.

- Evening activity: Have a history and trivia session on Chinese New Year. You can obtain information on Chinese New Year by researching the Internet ahead of time. For a fun way to end the activity, serve fortune cookies and Chinese tea. Have everyone read his or her fortune aloud. Play Chinese music during the gathering. This activity can accommodate any group size, and also can be done one-on-one in residents' rooms.

- Offer a Chinese cooking class during which residents prepare and enjoy an authentic Chinese meal together. Play Chinese music in the background. You will need to discuss the menu with residents ahead of time, decide on recipes, and purchase or secure all the supplies you'll need prior to the event. This activity can be held during either lunch or supper. It's best to keep this activity limited to only a small group.

For each activity, always welcome everyone to the group and always close the activity with a "Goodbye" and "See you next time." Praise and thank everyone for their participation.

Variations/adaptations/modifications: Some of the activities may be offered one-on-one for residents who are unwilling or unable to participate in a group. You will need to simplify tasks, make adaptations (some residents may not have the dexterity to fold paper, but may be able to choose the project and color of paper used), and offer more assistance to those residents with diminished abilities (some may be able to do some paper-folding with direct hand-over-hand guidance, whereas others may need additional verbal and visual cueing). Some activities can include low-functioning residents when adaptations/modifications are made.

Helpful hints/notes: Decorate the dining and activity areas in a Chinese New Year theme. Observe all infection-control guidelines and individual resident dietary needs/restrictions when serving food and beverages. You must know of any food allergies your residents may have, as many people are allergic to MSG, which is used in some Chinese food. For the origami activity, prepare and set up as much of the craft as possible ahead of time so that once residents are gathered you can begin the activity. Have an example for residents to see. Have all materials organized and direct residents throughout the program. Provide them with choices. Much of the setup for the cooking class can also be done prior to gathering residents so that you are ready to begin once residents have gathered. Assemble all needed equipment and supplies prior to the start of each activity. For the trivia game, encourage a positive atmosphere for fair, fun recreational play and competition. Announce and congratulate winners and players. Watch for signs of residents becoming overly tired or too competitive. Save all the information you've gathered for this event, laminate it or put it in plastic sleeves, and place it in a binder or folder labeled "Chinese New Year," and you now have an annual event already planned for years to come.

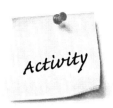

Activity | Christmas Charades

Target audience: Residents who enjoy social opportunities and acting, based on resident interests and needs

Objectives/outcomes:

- Promotes social interaction between peers and the staff

- Provides for companionship and conversation

- Promotes reminiscence, memory recall, mental stimulation, long-term memory skills, and cognitive/thinking skills

- Provides opportunities for recognition and builds self-esteem

Recommended group size: Medium

Suggested time frame: One hour

Special needs/ability level (physical/cognitive skills needed): Primarily residents with moderate to high cognitive functioning. Ability to follow directions, complete tasks, respond verbally, and interact on some level. Ability to read and act out words; requires cognitive reasoning skills. Because the words often draw on long-term memory, residents with moderate cognitive impairments can do surprisingly well with charades.

Activity outline:

- Prepare your Christmas charade words ahead of time by copying the words found on the file labeled Christmas Charades on your CD-ROM, laminating them, and then cutting them out with a paper cutter. Save them in a large manila envelope.

- Place the words face down in a basket.

- Ask a resident to volunteer to go first by picking a card. He or she then needs to act out that word. The staff can help a resident if the resident is unable to think of how to act out the word he or she has chosen, but be sure to give the resident time and encourage him or her to do it without staff assistance. The staff may also want to demonstrate one word first in case any residents don't understand the rules.

- Whoever guesses correctly first gets to pick the next word, and so on. If the same residents keep winning turns, you will need to let other residents have a turn before the end of the game.

Welcome everyone to the group and always close the activity with a "Goodbye" and "See you next time." Praise and thank everyone for their participation.

Variations/adaptations/modifications: Staff can come up with their own words based on different themes.

Helpful hints/notes: Much of the setup for this event can be done prior to gathering residents so that you are ready to begin once residents have gathered. Assemble all needed equipment and supplies prior to the start of the activity.

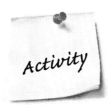

Activity | Cruise Week

Target audience: Residents who enjoy social opportunities, friendly competition, those who traveled and those who wished they could travel, based on resident interests and needs

Objectives/outcomes:

- Promotes social interaction among peers, family members, and the staff.

- Provides for companionship and conversation.

- Promotes reminiscence, mental stimulation, long-term memory skills, and cognitive/ thinking skills.

- Provides a learning opportunity.

- Provides opportunities for physical exercise and friendly competition in a recreational setting.

- Maintains and improves fine and gross motor skills.

- Maintains and improves hand-eye coordination.

- Develops a sense of pride and self-esteem associated with friendly competition and team play.

Recommended group size: Medium to large (varies based on activity)

Suggested time frame: 30 – 60 minutes for each activity

Special needs/ability level (physical/cognitive skills needed): Primarily residents with moderate to high cognitive functioning. Ability to follow directions, complete tasks, respond verbally, and interact on some level.

Activity outline:

- Map out your week of selected activities and cruise destinations (e.g., Alaska, Bermuda, the Bahamas and the Caribbean, Hawaii, Tahiti, Polynesia and the South Pacific, Northern Europe, Southern Europe, the Mediterranean, and Mexico). Make your cruise activities varied and exciting. Plan some specific activities that would be related to the areas you are visiting (dinners, entertainment, crafts, customs, etc.). Solicit posters, display ads, and so forth from travel agencies that they would otherwise just throw out. Make posters to advertise your upcoming cruise.

- Create a daily newspaper of activities and events that will occur the following day, and hand this out each afternoon so that residents can plan what they want to take part in the next day.

- Daytime activities can include exercise (yoga, tai chi, Pilates, tae kwon do, etc.; you can adapt the movements for all of these forms of exercise for residents who are wheelchair-bound), recreational games (shuffle board, ring toss, horseshoes, basketball, bowling, beanbag toss, etc.), wine tasting, demonstrations/classes (floral arranging, cake decorating, crafts, jewelry shows, kitchen demonstrations, home decorating demonstrations, etc.), theater shows (travel videos of your predetermined cruise destinations), and other organized activities.

- Plan day trips to shops, art galleries, museums, theaters, restaurants, and so on (depending on resident interests, cruise destination themes, and availability in your area).

- Nighttime activities can include a casino night (card games, keno, roulette, bingo, etc.), a live band/entertainment, a comedy show/gong show, karaoke, dance theater (local dance studios may come and perform), and so on.

- Offer a "spa," with open times for residents to visit throughout the week (so that they can get manicures, facials, and massages).

- Have a formal dinner with the "ship's captain" (the administrator).

For each activity, always welcome everyone to the group and always close the activity with a "Goodbye" and "See you next time." Praise and thank everyone for their participation.

Variations/adaptations/modifications: Some activities can be done on a one-on-one basis for those who cannot or will not take part in groups. You will need to simplify tasks, make adaptations (certain residents may need closer targets, or verbal and visual cues), and offer more assistance to residents with diminished abilities (they may be able to perform tasks with direct hand-over-hand guidance). Some activities can include low-functioning residents when adaptations/modifications are made.

Helpful hints/notes: Decorate the dining and activity areas with your selected cruise destination theme. Get the staff and residents' families involved in the events. Observe all infection-control guidelines and individual resident dietary needs/restrictions when serving food and beverages. Much of the setup for the event can be done prior to gathering residents so that you are ready to begin once residents have gathered. Assemble all needed equipment and supplies prior to the start of each activity. Encourage a positive atmosphere for fair, fun recreational play and competition. Save all of the information you have gathered for this event, laminate it or put it in plastic sleeves, and place it in a binder or folder labeled "Cruise Week," and you now have an annual event already planned for years to come.

Activity   Dairy Days Theme Week (June)

Target audience: Residents who enjoy social opportunities, especially those who farmed, based on resident interests and needs

Objectives/outcomes:

- Promotes social interaction between peers and the staff, mental stimulation, and recreation.

- Provides for companionship, refreshments, and conversation.

- Provides a learning opportunity.

- Butter or ice cream making: allows residents to express their creative ideas. Promotes residents' self-esteem through successful completion of projects. Maintains and develops fine motor skills and hand-eye coordination. Provides residents with an opportunity for choice and preference in regard to the finished project.

- Milk mustache contest, milking contest: provides opportunities for physical exercise and friendly competition in a recreational setting. To maintain and improve fine and gross motor skills. To maintain and improve hand-eye coordination. To develop a sense of pride and self-esteem associated with friendly competition and team play.

Recommended group size: Small or large (varies based on activity)

Suggested time frame: 30 – 60 minutes for each activity

Special needs/ability level (physical/cognitive skills needed): Primarily residents with moderate to high cognitive functioning. Ability to follow directions, complete tasks, respond verbally, and interact on some level.

Activity outline:

- Hold a milk mustache contest, which can include residents, volunteers, family members, and the staff. Do this activity on Monday through Thursday and hold the judging on Friday. Use either a digital or Polaroid camera. Use cream or buttermilk, as these are thicker and will stick to the upper lip. Seek contestants who desire to take part (always have residents' permission). Have contestants tip a glass of cream or buttermilk toward their closed lips so that the "milk" will stick to the upper lip. Take a picture of each contestant. Take pictures throughout the week and number and post them on a bulletin board in a highly visible area. You will need to have your "milk" on hand, as well as disposable Dixie cups and camera/film, throughout the week. On Friday, ask residents, volunteers, family members, and staff members to cast their vote by ballot, or by placing the number from the picture of the person they feel has the best "milk" mustache on a slip of paper and putting it in the ballot box. Announce the date, time, and location of the judging during the Monday through Thursday event, and erect a sign with this information in a visible area. Count the votes and announce the winner to the assembled group (also place the winner's name and photo on the bulletin board/display for all to see). Award an appropriate prize (this could be a food item, stuffed cow, etc.). This activity can accommodate any group size, and can be done one-on-one in residents' rooms (pictures of contestants and voting).

- Hold a cheese-tasting social. This is a great afternoon activity. Have a variety of cheeses and crackers for residents to sample. Serve regular milk and chocolate milk. Promote conversations with open-ended questions and encourage peer conversations. Tell residents to note the different textures and strengths of the various cheeses and discuss what they like and dislike about each. Discuss how cheese is made (you can get this information from the Internet). Play some background music of the residents' choosing. Usually this activity can accommodate a large group, but you also can conduct this activity with a small group on individual units.

- Have a butter-making activity. Get a butter recipe off the Internet or from a resident who may have made it in the past. Discuss the differences and myths between butter and margarine. Bake some biscuits and serve them warm, with the homemade butter. It's best to conduct this activity with a small group.

- Have a yogurt, malted milk, and black cow social on three different afternoons. For the yogurt social, offer residents a variety of different flavors to sample. You can also include frozen yogurt. For the malted milk social, make the malted milks with the residents in attendance, and serve them immediately before they get soupy. You can predetermine one flavor or offer a variety of flavors. For the black cow social (root beer and vanilla ice cream), make them in the residents' presence and serve them immediately before they get soupy. Play background music of the residents' choosing. Promote conversations with open-ended questions and encourage peer conversations. These are generally large group activities, but you can hold them in small groups on individual units, or as a "Treat Cart" where you go from room to room for those who cannot or will not attend group activities (but you lose the socialization aspect if you do it this way).

- Have a dairy days trivia contest. You can get your trivia from the Internet or from the Wisconsin Milk Marketing Board Web site (*http://producer.wisdairy.com/*), which offers recipes, dairy information, activity ideas, dairy statistics and trivia, and more). This activity can be held in a small or large group, and can be done one-on-one in residents' rooms.

- Visit a farm, or take a country ride by residents' old homesteads. You will need to coordinate any farm visits with the farmer (be sure the barn can accommodate wheelchairs), and have enough staff members or volunteers available to escort residents one-on-one. For a country ride, preselect residents who farmed and get directions to their farms so that you can drive by. (The men will love to see their old homestead.) You can stop at an ice cream shop and get ice cream cones for each resident on the bus as a treat.

- Have an ice cream making session. This is best done in a small or medium-size group, depending on the recipe and method you use to make the ice cream. If you're using a hand-crank ice cream maker (this is the method I prefer as it gets the residents physically involved and you can have a discussion group while making the ice cream), here is a sample recipe:

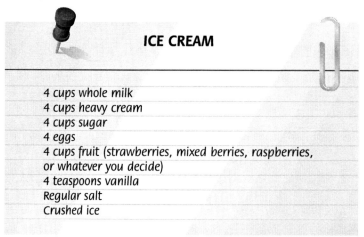

ICE CREAM

4 cups whole milk
4 cups heavy cream
4 cups sugar
4 eggs
4 cups fruit (strawberries, mixed berries, raspberries, or whatever you decide)
4 teaspoons vanilla
Regular salt
Crushed ice

- Place milk, cream, sugar, eggs (slightly beaten), and vanilla inside the ice cream container. Place the container inside the wooden ice cream maker and secure the crank handle. Fill the sides with crushed ice and pour salt over the crushed ice. Have residents take turns cranking the handle. You will need to add additional ice and salt throughout the process. Crank steadily for 45 minutes. Remove the inside container from the ice cream maker and wipe it down to get the salt off the outside of the container. Open the container and add the fruit. I have found it's best to add the fruit after the ice cream is made as you will get a thicker consistency this way and the fruit will not freeze as it does when you add it in the beginning with the other ingredients. Serve and enjoy! (We have done this for 15 years and have never had anyone get sick from the raw eggs in the ice cream.) This recipe is high in sugar and calories and is very rich, so small portions are best, and very small portions are best for diabetics.

- Hold a "milking" contest. Poke pinholes into the fingers and thumbs of a pair of rubber gloves (more than one hole in each). Fill with milk. Tie the top of the gloves in a knot as you would a balloon. Suspend the gloves with a piece of string in a row from a portable coat rack so that they hang down. Have buckets underneath to milk into. Have contestants line up, and when you give the signal, have them "milk" their gloves. The person to get the most milk into the bucket wins. This will generate a lot of laughs from those watching and participating. They will need good hand dexterity to have any success at milking.

- Have an ice cream social (we cover this in Chapter 12).

For each activity, always welcome everyone to the group and always close the activity with a "Goodbye" and "See you next time." Praise and thank everyone for their participation.

Variations/adaptations/modifications: Some of these activities may be offered one-on-one with residents who are unwilling or unable to participate in a group. You will need to simplify tasks, make adaptations (certain residents may need closer targets, or verbal and visual cues), and offer more assistance to those residents with diminished abilities (they may be able to perform tasks with direct hand-over-hand guidance). Some activities can include low-functioning residents when adaptations/modifications are made.

Helpful hints/notes: Decorate the dining and activity areas in a "dairy days" theme. Observe all infection-control guidelines and individual resident dietary needs/restrictions when serving food and beverages. You must know of any food allergies your residents may have. Much of the setup for these events can be done prior to gathering residents so that you are ready to begin once residents have gathered. Assemble all needed equipment and supplies prior to the start of each activity. Encourage a positive atmosphere for fair, fun recreational play and competition. Announce and congratulate winners and players. Watch for signs of any residents becoming overly tired or too competitive. Save all the information you've gathered for this event, laminate it or put it in plastic sleeves, and place it in a binder or folder labeled "Dairy Days Week," and you now have an annual event already planned for years to come.

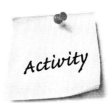 **Activity** | **Folk Fair**

Target audience: Residents who enjoy social opportunities, based on resident interests and needs, especially residents who enjoy cultural activities

Objectives/outcomes:

- Promotes social interaction between peers and the staff, mental stimulation, and recreation

- Provides for companionship, refreshments, and conversation

- Provides a learning opportunity

- Provides an opportunity for reminiscence, which promotes mental stimulation, long-term memory skills, and cognitive/thinking skills

Recommended group size: Five or six at each booth at any given time is best

Suggested time frame: Ninety minutes to allow residents to visit each booth

Special needs/ability level (physical/cognitive skills needed): All residents can participate on some level. Moderately impaired residents may need verbal and visual cues and direct physical guidance. Severely impaired residents may enjoy observing demonstrations and viewing finished products.

Activity outline:

- Contact your local senior center to see whether they are able to help you set up this program. Often, senior centers conduct folk fairs for grade school classes and can easily conduct a folk fair for your residents. Usually they will do this program for free. Otherwise, you will need to find people in your community and make the contacts yourself for the various booths. Once you do the initial legwork, this is a great program to offer on an annual basis.

- You will need adequate space to set up the different booths for residents to stop by and visit. Your available space and the needs of the exhibitors will determine how many booths you can set up. Usually each exhibitor wants an 8-foot table and a few chairs, but you will need to know this in advance so that you can have the room set up prior to their arrival. Plan to allow them 30 minutes (or more) to set up and take down their exhibits after the event.

- You will need an adequate staff and/or volunteers to assist all residents who need assistance getting to the different booths. Residents usually will spend 10 to 15 minutes at each booth; again, this will vary according to what is being demonstrated and the individual interests of each resident. Some residents may go back several times to any number of booths if they find something particularly interesting.

- Advertise your event ahead of time to encourage residents' family members to attend. This makes it easier for the staff and/or volunteers to focus on residents without family present.

- Here are some suggested exhibitors to seek out (these are appropriate to our area and the cultural backgrounds of the majority of our residents): bee keeping (demonstration and honey tasting), wood carving (demonstration and finished products to view), wood working (demonstration and finished products to view), butter making (offer free tasting and let residents take part at this booth), ice cream making (offer free tasting and let residents take part at this booth), weaving (demonstration and finished products to view), spinning wool (demonstration and finished products to view), rag rug making (demonstration and finished products to view), doll making (demonstration and finished products to view), doll house making (demonstration and finished product to view), jewelry making/beading (demonstration and finished products to view), and quilting (demonstration and finished products to view). Of course, there are many others to be considered as well.

- Promote resident reminiscing as they visit each booth. Don't forget to take lots of candid camera shots to capture those special moments of joy.

- Play background folk music.

Variations/adaptations/modifications: For low-functioning residents, bring the props closer and allow them to touch, hold, and feel the different items as you talk to them about the items and the various textures they are feeling.

Helpful hints/notes: Observe all infection-control guidelines and individual resident dietary needs/restrictions when serving food and beverages. Much of the setup for this event can be done prior to gathering residents so that you are ready to begin once residents have gathered. Assemble all needed equipment and supplies prior to the start of the activity. Save all the information you've gathered for this event, laminate it or put it in plastic sleeves, and place it in a binder or folder labeled "Folk Fair," and you now have an annual event already planned for years to come.

Gay '90s Luncheon

Target audience: Residents who are 90 years of age and older

Objectives/outcomes:

- Promotes social interaction between peers and the staff

- Provides for companionship, refreshments, and conversation

- Provides an opportunity for reminiscence, which promotes mental stimulation, long-term memory skills, and cognitive/thinking skills

- Promotes a positive self-esteem and provides recognition

Recommended group size: Varies by number of residents 90 years of age and older

Suggested time frame: 60 – 90 minutes

Special needs/ability level (physical/cognitive skills needed): Primarily residents with moderate to high cognitive functioning. You must be able to accommodate residents' dietary needs within the setting.

Activity outline:

- Have the Dietary Department plan a special lunch menu and serve it in a separate dining area/activity area for just the special guests. Or have a special meal catered in. Serve "birthday cake" for dessert. Promote conversations with open-ended questions and encourage peer conversations, especially about all the changes they have seen in their lifetime. Play background dinner music to set the mood, and to develop a pleasant and appropriate celebratory atmosphere.

- Have a musician play prior to the meal or after the meal. Selection of the musician should be based on residents' music preference (e.g., sing-along, guitar, piano, concertina, etc.). Make sure that "Happy Birthday" is played and sung by all in attendance.

- At some point in the event, with the residents' permission, ask which residents in attendance are the oldest and youngest. Make them all feel honored and special to have achieved such a milestone of being 90 or older.

- Give corsages to all the celebrants as they arrive at the event.

For each activity, always welcome everyone to the group and always close the activity with a "Goodbye" and "See you next time." Praise and thank everyone for their participation.

Variations/adaptations/modifications: Allow residents to invite a guest to accompany them to this event for a nominal fee, or for free if your budget allows.

Helpful hints/notes: Decorate the area in a birthday party theme. Encourage residents to dress up for the party. Observe all infection-control guidelines and individual resident dietary needs/restrictions when serving food and beverages. Much of the setup for this event can be done prior to gathering residents so that you are ready to begin once residents have gathered. Assemble all needed equipment and supplies prior to the start of the activity.

Grandparents' Day Party

Target audience: Residents who enjoy social opportunities, based on resident interests and needs, especially residents who have grandchildren or great-grandchildren or who just enjoy children in general

Objectives/outcomes:

- Promotes social interaction and recognition among peers, family members, and children

- Provides for companionship, refreshments, and conversation

- Provides an opportunity for reminiscence, which promotes mental stimulation, long-term memory skills, and cognitive/thinking skills

Recommended group size: Large

Suggested time frame: From one to two hours

Special needs/ability level (physical/cognitive skills needed): All residents can participate on some level, even if it's just to observe the environment.

Activity outline:

- Advertise a "Grandparents' Day" party and invite residents' grandchildren and great-grandchildren. You may want to include staff grandchildren for residents who do not have any.

- Schedule a band to play music that a majority of your residents like. Encourage the children to dance with grandma and grandpa. Don't forget the hokey pokey and the chicken dance.

- Serve refreshments. Cookies and punch work well.

- Promote interaction between children and residents.

- Take pictures of grandparents and grandchildren and give a copy to each.

Variations/adaptations/modifications: Instead of having a band, you could play recreational games (e.g., ring toss, basketball, beanbag toss, fishing [offer prizes for the children], or bingo), and serve refreshments as a conclusion to the games.

Helpful hints/notes: Observe all infection-control guidelines and individual resident dietary needs/restrictions when serving food and beverages. Much of the setup for this event can be done prior to gathering residents so that you are ready to begin once residents have gathered. Assemble all needed equipment and supplies prior to the start of the activity.

Halloween Party

Target audience: Residents who enjoy social opportunities and friendly competition, based on resident interests and needs

Objectives/outcomes:

- Promotes social interaction among peers, family members, and the staff

- Provides for companionship and conversation

- Promotes reminiscence and humor

- Provides opportunities for friendly competition in a social setting

Recommended group size: Large

Suggested time frame: One hour

Special needs/ability level (physical/cognitive skills needed): All residents can participate on some level.

Activity outline:

- Hold a resident and staff costume contest. Provide or encourage residents' families to provide costumes. The staff should dress residents in the morning in their costumes, only with resident permission, of course. Caution: *Do not* have a confused male resident dress as a female or vice versa, as you cannot know or get his or her permission to do so and this could be upsetting to family members. Always maintain resident dignity. In the morning at a predetermined time, schedule pictures to be taken of the residents and the staff, and number and place the photos on a poster. Display the poster in a prominent area and have the residents and staff vote for best costume based on the number on the picture. Allow only one vote per resident and staff member.

- Hold the Halloween party in the afternoon (or evening), and midway through have a "Parade of Costumes" and then announce the winner of the costume contest (give a prize to the declared winner; a Halloween or fall item is a good choice). For the party, either schedule an entertainer or band based on resident music preference, or perform a Halloween skit. The song "The Monster Mash" is easy to do a skit to, it's fun and humorous, it's guaranteed to generate a lot of laughs, and you really don't have to put in much practice time as spontaneity is all the better.

- Serve Halloween cookies and orange punch. In the party area, set up a witch's cauldron with dry ice, which will make it look like "witches' brew," and use a fog machine.

For this activity, always welcome everyone to the group and always close the activity with a "Goodbye" and "See you next time." Praise and thank everyone for their participation.

Variations/adaptations/modifications: Some activities can be done on a one-on-one basis for those who cannot or will not take part in groups. Have a cookie baking and decorating session in the morning for refreshments to be served later in the day for the party. You can make and serve "worm dirt cake" (chocolate cake with brown frosting and sprinkles, with gummy worms on top). You can float peeled grapes in punch for "eyeball punch." As part of the party (and for one-on-one visits), place peeled grapes (eyeballs), green Jell-o (ghost guts), large dog biscuits (human bones), and cooked spaghetti that has congealed overnight (human brain) in plastic bags inside brown paper bags. Have residents reach in and feel the contents. Watch and capture reactions on film; it is hilarious and most residents really enjoy this fun sensory experience. (Do this only with their permission, of course.) After everyone has had a chance to feel the contents of each bag, show them what was really in the bags. Some will have been able to guess correctly. Have a "bobbing for donuts" contest. Suspend donuts with yarn from a coat rack at the level of residents' mouths. Solicit residents who want to take part and pair residents with similar abilities to have a friendly contest against each other one-on-one. The object is to be the first to bite a chunk out of the donut; residents can only use their mouths, not their hands. (Of course, they get an extra treat as they get their donuts at the completion of their contest. Have a dozen or more donuts on hand to allow as many residents to take part as time allows.) This generates a lot of laughs, too. Capture the moments on film. Schedule a Halloween trick or treat with staff members' children in the afternoon or evening. Have them go up and down the halls/units. Provide residents with candy to hand out to the visiting children who are in costume.

Helpful hints/notes: Decorate the dining and activity areas in a Halloween theme. Get all staff members and residents' families involved in the events. Much of the setup for these events can be done prior to gathering residents so that you are ready to begin once residents have gathered. Observe all infection-control guidelines and individual resident dietary needs/restrictions when serving food and beverages. Assemble all needed equipment and supplies prior to the start of each activity.

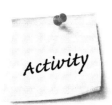

Activity | **Mardi Gras Theme Day**

Target audience: Residents who enjoy social opportunities, based on resident interests and needs

Objectives/outcomes:

- Promotes social interaction between peers and the staff, mental stimulation, and recreation.

- Provides for companionship, refreshments, and conversation.

- Provides a cultural and learning opportunity.

- Cooking class: allows residents to express their creative ideas. Promotes residents' self-esteem through successful completion of projects. Maintains and develops fine motor skills and hand-eye coordination. Provides residents with an opportunity for choice and preference in regard to the finished project.

- Recreational games: provide opportunities for exercise and friendly competition in a recreational setting. To maintain and improve fine and gross motor skills. To maintain and improve hand-eye coordination. To develop a sense of pride and self-esteem associated with friendly competition and team play. To provide opportunities for mild cardiovascular stimulation.

Recommended group size: Small or large (varies based on activity)

Suggested time frame: 30 – 60 minutes for each activity

Special needs/ability level (physical/cognitive skills needed): Primarily residents with moderate to high cognitive functioning. Ability to follow directions, complete tasks, respond verbally, and interact on some level.

Activity outline:

- Morning activity: Have a Mardi Gras history and trivia session. You can obtain the history and trivia information by researching the subject on the Internet ahead of time. Play Mardi Gras music while gathering and assisting residents to and from the activity. This activity can accommodate any group size and also can be done one-on-one in rooms.

- Luncheon activity: Have the Dietary Department prepare a Mardi Gras dinner for all residents. Play Mardi Gras music to set the mood (in all dining areas), and to develop a pleasant and appropriate atmosphere. Promote conversations with open-ended questions and encourage peer conversations.

- Evening activity: Have a Mardi Gras parade. Have residents dress in Mardi Gras colors of gold, green, and purple for the day. Purchase Mardi Gras masks and gold, green, and purple beads for residents to wear (from a party supply store/catalog). Have the staff, residents' family members, and volunteers "parade" the residents down the halls to the activity area. Once there, form a big circle around the perimeter (you may have to form a double circle depending on the size of the room). Have Mardi Gras music playing. Have the "crowd/residents" shout, "Show some leg," and whenever someone shows some leg that person gets a string of beads thrown to him or her to add to his or her collection. Whoever gets the most beads could be awarded a prize of something that goes with the theme. Next, move on to a coin toss game. You can purchase gold, green, and purple coins from a party supply store or catalog. Have residents take turns tossing coins into a bucket or pot (decide ahead of time how many coins each resident will receive). Whoever gets the most coins into the bucket/pot wins a prize (make the prize something that goes with the theme, which you will have had to purchase ahead of time). Lastly, serve "king cake" or some other Creole or Cajun snack and grape juice or green Kool-Aid (for the purple or green beverage).

- Offer a Creole or Cajun cooking class where residents prepare and enjoy an authentic Creole/Cajun meal together. Play Mardi Gras music in the background. You will need to discuss the menu with the residents ahead of time, decide on recipes, and purchase or secure the necessary supplies prior to the event. This could be either a lunch or a supper event. This activity is best kept to a small group.

- Have a pancake breakfast (or supper). Have the Activities Department along with the administrator make breakfast/supper (pancakes) for the residents that day, and serve the pancakes hot off the griddle. Have the dietary staff prepare the pancake batter and the rest of the breakfast/supper menu.

- Have a "flying flapjack" contest as the morning or afternoon activity. Use foam Frisbees and have residents aim at a target (either a line across the floor or a basket to toss them into). Allow each resident a predetermined number of tries. The resident with the most targets wins a prize (something that goes with the theme).

For each activity, always welcome everyone to the group and always close the activity with a "Goodbye" and "See you next time." Praise and thank everyone for their participation.

Variations/adaptations/modifications: Some of the activities may be offered one-on-one with residents who are unwilling or unable to participate in a group. You will need to simplify tasks, make adaptations (certain residents may need closer targets for some of the games, or verbal and visual cues), and offer more assistance to residents with diminished abilities (they may be able to perform tasks with direct hand-over-hand guidance). Some activities can include low-functioning residents when adaptations/modifications are made.

Helpful hints/notes: Decorate the dining and activity areas in a Mardi Gras theme. Observe all infection-control guidelines and individual resident dietary needs/restrictions when serving food and beverages. You must know of any food allergies your residents may have. Much of the setup for the cooking class can be done prior to gathering residents so that you are ready to begin once residents have gathered. Assemble all needed equipment and supplies prior to the start of each activity. Encourage a positive atmosphere for fair, fun recreational play and competition. Announce and congratulate winners and players. Watch for signs of any residents becoming overly tired or too competitive. Save all the information you've gathered for this event, laminate it or put it in plastic sleeves, and place it in a binder or folder labeled "Mardi Gras," and you now have an annual event already planned for years to come.

Mexican Fiesta Day

Target audience: Residents who enjoy social opportunities, based on resident interests and needs

Objectives/outcomes:

- Promotes social interaction between peers and the staff, mental stimulation, and recreation.

- Provides for companionship, refreshments, and conversation.

- Provides a learning opportunity.

- Piñata game and exercises: provide opportunities for physical exercise and friendly competition in a recreational setting. To maintain and improve fine and gross motor skills. To maintain and improve hand-eye coordination. To develop a sense of pride and self-esteem associated with friendly competition and team play.

- Cooking class: allows residents to express their creative ideas. Promotes residents' self-esteem through successful completion of projects. Maintains and develops fine motor skills and hand-eye coordination. Provides residents with an opportunity for choice and preference in regard to the finished project.

Recommended group size: Small or large (varies based on activity)

Suggested time frame: 30 – 60 minutes for each activity

Special needs/ability level (physical/cognitive skills needed): Primarily residents with moderate to high cognitive functioning. Ability to follow directions, complete tasks, respond verbally, and interact on some level.

Activity outline:

- Have the Dietary Department plan a Mexican dinner for all residents. Promote conversations with open-ended questions and encourage peer conversations. Play background Mexican/mariachi music to set the mood (in all dining areas), and to develop a pleasant and appropriate atmosphere.

- Have an outing to a Mexican restaurant.

- Offer a Mexican cooking class where residents prepare and enjoy an authentic Mexican meal together. Play Mexican/mariachi music in the background. You will need to discuss the menu with the residents ahead of time, decide on recipes, and purchase or secure the necessary supplies prior to the event. This could be either a lunch or a supper event. This activity is best kept to a small group.

- Conduct morning exercises set to Mexican/mariachi music, using mariachis and clappers (you can also utilize other rhythm instruments) and colorful scarves. Have residents move their arms and legs to the music.

- For an afternoon event, fill a piñata with candy and hang it from the ceiling. Have residents swing at it blindfolded (use the colorful scarves from the morning activity; each resident should have his or her own clean scarf for infection control purposes) with a plastic bat. You will need to provide them with verbal clues and set them up in front of the piñata. Keep residents safe at all times by monitoring the group and not letting the bat make contact with anything other than the piñata. Once the piñata breaks, everyone can take some candy. Play Mexican/mariachi music in the background during this activity.

- Have a margarita social. You can offer one flavor or a variety of flavors. Be sure to make the margaritas in the residents' presence and serve the margaritas immediately so they are nice and frozen. Serve chips and salsa. Play background Mexican/mariachi music. Promote conversations with open-ended questions and encourage peer conversations. This is generally a large group activity, but you can hold this activity for small groups on individual units or in the form of a "Treat Cart" whereby you visit each resident in his or her room (although this latter approach is good for residents who cannot or will not attend group activities, you will lose the socialization aspect doing it this way).

For each activity, always welcome everyone to the group and always close the activity with a "Goodbye" and "See you next time." Praise and thank everyone for their participation.

Variations/adaptations/modifications: Some of the activities may be offered one-on-one with residents who are unwilling or unable to participate in a group. You will need to simplify tasks, make adaptations (certain residents may need closer targets, or verbal and visual cues), and offer more assistance to those residents with diminished abilities (they may be able to perform tasks with direct hand-over-hand guidance). Some activities can include low-functioning residents when adaptations/modifications are made.

Helpful hints/notes: Decorate the dining and activity areas in a Mexican theme. Encourage residents and the staff to dress in Mexican attire (or in bright/festive colors) for the day. Observe all infection-control guidelines and individual resident dietary needs/restrictions when serving food and beverages. You must know of any food allergies your residents may have. Much of the setup for these events can be done prior to gathering residents so that you are ready to begin once residents have gathered. Assemble all needed equipment and supplies prior to the start of each activity. Encourage a positive atmosphere for fair, fun recreational play and competition. Announce and congratulate winners and players. Watch for signs of any residents becoming overly tired or too competitive. Save all the information you've gathered for this event, laminate it or put it in plastic sleeves, and place it in a binder or folder labeled "Mexican Fiesta Day," and you now have an annual event already planned for years to come.

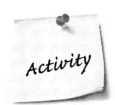

Activity | New Year's Celebration

Target audience: Residents who enjoy social opportunities, based on resident interests and needs

Objectives/outcomes:

- Promotes social interaction between peers and the staff

- Provides for companionship, refreshments, and conversation

- Promotes reminiscence

Recommended group size: Medium to large

Suggested time frame: One hour

Special needs/ability level (physical/cognitive skills needed): All residents can take part on some level.

Activity outline:

- Schedule a band or musician to play music that most of your residents like.

- Pass out New Year's hats, noisemakers, horns, and leis.

- Serve hors d'oeuvres and champagne in champagne glasses (offer nonalcoholic drinks as well). Say a New Year's toast for all in attendance.

- Count down from 10 to one (at which point you could have balloons/confetti drop from the ceiling), have everyone shout "Happy New Year," and have the band play "Auld Lang Syne."

For each activity, always welcome everyone to the group and always close the activity with a "Goodbye" and "See you next time." Praise and thank everyone for their participation.

Helpful hints/notes: Observe all infection-control guidelines and individual resident dietary needs/restrictions when serving food and beverages. Much of the setup for this event can be done prior to gathering residents so that you are ready to begin once residents have gathered. Assemble all needed equipment and supplies prior to the start of the activity.

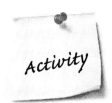

Activity   **President's Day Silhouettes**

Target audience: Residents who enjoy social opportunities, based on resident interests and needs

Objectives/outcomes:

- Promotes social interaction among peers, family members, and the staff

- Provides for companionship and conversation

- Promotes reminiscence, mental stimulation, long-term memory skills, and cognitive/ thinking skills

- Promotes residents' self-esteem through successful projects

Recommended group size: Small to medium

Suggested time frame: One hour

Special needs/ability level (physical/cognitive skills needed): Primarily residents with moderate to high cognitive functioning. Residents need to be able to sit up straight in a chair and hold their position for several minutes. If they can do that, they can participate.

Activity outline:

- You will need black and white construction paper, an overhead projector, a spot light or flash light, and pencils for tracing.

- Begin with a short discussion about the famous president silhouettes of Lincoln and Washington (show them samples). Explain that they are going to be famous too with the "Wall of Fame of Residents of [your facility name]."

- Have each resident in attendance have his or her silhouette drawn. Tape a piece of construction paper (either black or white) to the wall, have each resident sit sideways in front of the paper so that his or her head and neck reflect onto the paper when a light is shone on it. Trace the resident's silhouette onto the paper. While you move on to the next resident, other staff members can be cutting out the silhouettes and placing them onto a piece of paper the opposite color of the one you used.

- Put residents' names on the back of each silhouette and tape them to a poster titled "Residents' Wall of Fame." Place the poster in a prominent area so that everyone can see it. Staff members, residents, and families will have a fun time guessing who is who. Residents will take pride in taking their family members to the Wall of Fame and pointing themselves out. Leave the display up for at least a month; then take it down and give each resident his or her silhouette to keep. (You will be surprised how easy it is to tell who is who.)

For each activity, always welcome everyone to the group and always close the activity with a "Goodbye" and "See you next time." Praise and thank everyone for their participation.

Variations/adaptations/modifications: It may be possible to do this activity one-on-one in residents' rooms for those who cannot or will not participate in groups. That way, every resident can be included on the Wall of Fame. You could hold a trivia/discussion group in the morning about presidents and pique residents' interest in the afternoon activity, but don't divulge what you plan to do. Just tell them that if they want to be famous, they should come down this afternoon to learn about the Wall of Fame.

Helpful hints/notes: Much of the setup for this event can be done prior to gathering residents so that you are ready to begin once residents have gathered. Assemble all needed equipment and supplies prior to the start of the activity.

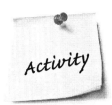

Resident Academy Awards

Target audience: Residents who enjoy social opportunities and recognition, based on resident interests and needs

Objectives/outcomes:

- Promotes social interaction among peers, family members, and the staff

- Provides for companionship and conversation

- Promotes reminiscence

- Provides opportunities for recognition and builds self-esteem

Recommended group size: Varies

Suggested time frame: One hour

Special needs/ability level (physical/cognitive skills needed): All residents can participate on some level.

Activity outline:

- Schedule a "Resident Academy Awards" event during a special week, such as Nursing Home Week or in conjunction with the Academy Awards.

- Advertise the event with posters and invite residents' family members to attend. Encourage all staff members to attend as well. Build up the hype.

- Have all staff members nominate a resident to receive an award using a ballot form located on the CD-ROM. You, as the activities director, will have to make sure every resident receives an Academy Award for something.

- Encourage everyone to dress in their Sunday best for the event. Or, residents can wear gowns and suits if they have them.

- The activities director can be the host of the event and the administrator can hand out the awards. The suggested attire can be formal wear. As the host, you will announce each award and the nominees, followed by the winner of the award. Make everyone feel special, and highlight why each individual won his or her particular award. Have volunteers/family members/staff members on hand to escort the residents to receive their awards. Take a picture of each resident as he or she receives an award and display the photos in a prominent area following the ceremony. (Make award certificates ahead of time and have them ready to hand out during the event; a template is located on the CD-ROM. Either create a certificate on the computer or purchase certificate paper onto which you can copy the awards.

- Serve refreshments following the awards presentation. Serve champagne (rent a champagne fountain), chocolate fondue (rent a fondue fountain), or other gourmet refreshments.

For each activity, always welcome everyone to the group and always close the activity with a "Goodbye" and "See you next time." Praise and thank everyone for their participation.

Variations/adaptations/modifications: Some activities can be done on a one-on-one basis for those who cannot or will not take part in groups (e.g., present their awards individually in their rooms and take their pictures as well).

Helpful hints/notes: Decorate the activity area in an Academy Awards theme (roll out the red carpet). Observe all infection-control guidelines and individual resident dietary needs/restrictions when serving food and beverages. Much of the setup for this event can be done prior to gathering residents so that you are ready to begin once residents have gathered. Assemble all needed equipment and supplies prior to the start of this activity. Save all the information you've gathered for this event, laminate it or put it in plastic sleeves, and place it in a binder or folder labeled "Resident Academy Awards," and you now have an annual event already planned for years to come.

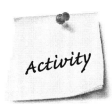

Activity | **Senior Prom**

Target audience: Residents who enjoy social opportunities and recognition, based on resident interests and needs

Objectives/outcomes:

- Promotes social interaction among peers, family members, students, and staff members

- Provides for companionship and conversation

- Promotes reminiscence

- Provides opportunities for recognition and builds self-esteem

Recommended group size: Varies

Suggested time frame: 60 – 90 minutes

Special needs/ability level (physical/cognitive skills needed): All residents can participate on some level.

Activity outline:

- Seek a high school group such as the National Honor Society to have a senior prom with your residents one or two weeks following the high school prom (which usually takes place in April or May). Students should come dressed in their prom attire.

- Schedule a band or deejay (to play residents' musical preferences, as well as some good dance music). This will need to be an evening activity.

- Advertise the event with posters and invite residents' family members to attend. Encourage all staff members to attend as well. Build up the hype.

- Encourage everyone to dress up for the event.

- Have the Dietary Department plan a special evening meal, such as chicken cordon bleu, shrimp, or steak. Have department heads dress in black and white and be the servers. Serve wine and a special dessert. Play background dinner music.

- Have a corsage/boutonnière for each resident and pin it on as they are escorted to the prom by the students/staff. Take pictures.

- The students should dance with the residents. Include the bunny hop, hokey pokey, and chicken dance and encourage residents to join in as they are able.

- Crown a prom king and queen. (Have the students select the prom king and queen, or have the residents select a prom king and queen ahead of time.) Have a special dance just for them.

- Serve punch and cookies.

For each activity, always welcome everyone to the group and always close the activity with a "Goodbye" and "See you next time." Praise and thank everyone for their participation.

Variations/adaptations/modifications: See whether the school will help to offset the cost of entertainment, flowers, and refreshments.

Helpful hints/notes: Decorate the activity area in a prom theme (possibly the school's prom decorations could be used and students could decorate the area for you). Observe all infection-control guidelines and individual resident dietary needs/restrictions when serving food and beverages. Much of the setup for the event can be done prior to gathering residents so that you are ready to begin once residents have gathered. Assemble all needed equipment and supplies prior to the start of the activity. Save all the information you've gathered for this event, laminate it or put it in plastic sleeves, and place it in a binder or folder labeled "Senior Prom," and you now have an annual event already planned for years to come.

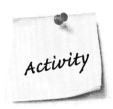

Activity

Spring Fling Party/Social

Target audience: Residents who enjoy social opportunities, reminiscing, and discussion, based on resident interests and needs

Objectives/outcomes:

- Promotes social interaction between peers and the staff

- Provides for companionship, refreshments, and conversation

Recommended group size: Medium to large

Suggested time frame: One hour

Special needs/ability level (physical/cognitive skills needed): All residents can take part on some level.

Activity outline:

- Schedule a band or musician to play music that the majority of your residents like.

- Make sure everyone knows you are saying goodbye to winter and celebrating the beginning of spring. (This is a good event for the first day of spring.) Encourage gaiety with singing, dancing, and movement to music.

- Serve rainbow sherbet.

For each activity, always welcome everyone to the group and always close the activity with a "Goodbye" and "See you next time." Praise and thank everyone for their participation.

Variations/adaptations/modifications: Hold a morning discussion group to set the festive mood for the "Spring Fling" later that day. Discuss/reminisce about spring, rebirth (baby animals, flowers blossoming, trees budding, etc.), spring cleaning, planning gardens, the changes in weather, and so on.

Helpful hints/notes: Decorate the area in a spring/Easter theme. Place tulips, hyacinths, and daffodils in vases/pots around the room; these can also be used for one-on-one, in-room sensory visits. Encourage everyone to wear brightly colored spring clothes for the day. Observe all infection-control guidelines and individual resident dietary needs/restrictions when serving food and beverages. Much of the setup for the event can be done prior to gathering residents so that you are ready to begin once residents have gathered. Assemble all needed equipment and supplies prior to the start of the activity.

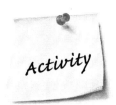

Activity

St. Patrick's Day Party/Social

Target audience: Residents who enjoy social opportunities, reminiscing, and discussion, based on resident interests and needs, especially those of Irish heritage

Objectives/outcomes:

- Promotes social interaction between peers and the staff

- Provides for companionship, refreshments, and conversation

- Provides an opportunity for reminiscence, which promotes mental stimulation, long-term memory skills, and cognitive/thinking skills

- Trivia/discussion groups: promote mental stimulation, long-term memory skills, and cognitive/thinking skills

Recommended group size: Medium to large

Suggested time frame: One hour

Special needs/ability level (physical/cognitive skills needed): All residents can take part on some level.

Activity outline:

- Play Irish music or have a band that can perform Irish songs.

- Encourage singing, dancing, and movement to music; try the Irish jig if you're brave.

- Discuss and share Irish blessings (use the Internet as your resource).

- Serve only "green" beverages and snacks (e.g., green beer if you have access [Wisconsin does], green Kool-Aid, pistachio dessert, green chips, green frosted shamrock cookies, shamrock shakes [crème de menthe topping] or grasshoppers [crème de menthe liquor blended with vanilla ice cream], mint ice cream, lime Jell-o, and so on).

For each activity, always welcome everyone to the group and always close the activity with a "Goodbye" and "See you next time." Praise and thank everyone for their participation.

Variations/adaptations/modifications: If music is not available, show a video of Ireland, have some Irish trivia, and serve only "green" snacks/beverages as noted above. You could also make Irish soda bread in a morning group and serve it at the afternoon gathering.

Helpful hints/notes: Decorate the area in a St. Patrick's Day theme. Encourage everyone to wear green for the day. You can also purchase hats, necklaces, and other Irish paraphernalia from a party supply store, dollar discount store, or catalog. This will help to make it a very festive party. You can reuse the decorations and other Irish paraphernalia from year to year. Observe all infection-control guidelines and individual resident dietary needs/restrictions when serving food and beverages. Much of the setup for the event can be done prior to gathering residents so that you are ready to begin once residents have gathered. Assemble all needed equipment and supplies prior to the start of the activity.

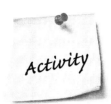

Activity | **Thanksgiving Blessings**

Target audience: Residents who enjoy social opportunities, reminiscing, and simple crafts, based on resident interests and needs

Objectives/outcomes:

- Promotes social interaction between peers and the staff

- Provides for companionship, refreshments, and conversation

- Provides a simple creative outlet and sense of pride

- Creates a sense of thankfulness/reminds others there is a lot to be thankful for

- Provides an opportunity for reminiscence, which promotes mental stimulation, long-term memory skills, and cognitive/thinking skills

- Trivia/discussion groups: promote mental stimulation, long-term memory skills, and cognitive/thinking skills

Recommended group size: Small to medium

Suggested time frame: One hour

Special needs/ability level (physical/cognitive skills needed): Primarily residents with moderate to high cognitive functioning. Ability to follow directions, complete tasks, respond verbally, and interact on some level.

Activity outline:

- You will need copy or construction paper in fall colors, black markers, yarn, and scissors. (Markers are easy to trace with and the lines are dark enough to see.)

- Let residents choose the color of paper they would like.

- Have each resident trace his or her hand on the paper.

- Have each resident cut out his or her hand shape.

- Discuss what blessings they have in their lives and encourage them to write at least one blessing on their paper hand. Have them sign their name on their paper hand.

- Attach all hands to a string (the string should be one continuous string, so the length of the string will depend on the number of participants).

- Display the "String of Blessings" in a prominent place where it can be viewed by all residents, staff members, and family members. Encourage residents to visit the "String of Blessings" when family members visit for Thanksgiving.

For each activity, always welcome everyone to the group and always close the activity with a "Goodbye" and "See you next time." Praise and thank everyone for their participation.

Variations/adaptations/modifications: May be offered one-on-one with residents who are unwilling or unable to participate in a group (you can simply add their paper hands to the string). You will need to simplify tasks, make adaptations (verbal and visual cues), and offer more assistance to those residents with diminished abilities (those who may be able to perform tasks with direct hand-over-hand guidance). Some activities can include low-functioning residents when adaptations/modifications are made. You may need to place a resident's hand onto the paper and trace it for him or her. You may need to cut out the paper hand and write the resident's name and blessing on it if the resident is unable to do this by him or herself. You could provide materials for staff and family members (and for residents who didn't initially take part) to add their blessings to the "String of Blessings" throughout the month and see how long you can get the string (make it a competition to see whether you can get it to go throughout the facility in 30 days).

Helpful hints/notes: Much of the setup for this event can be done prior to gathering residents so that you are ready to begin once residents have gathered. Assemble all needed equipment and supplies prior to the start of the activity.

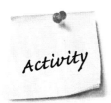

Activity

Thanksgiving Social

Target audience: Residents who enjoy social opportunities, reminiscing, and discussion, based on resident interests and needs

Objectives/outcomes:

- Promotes social interaction between peers and the staff

- Provides for companionship, refreshments, and conversation

- Provides an opportunity for reminiscence, which promotes mental stimulation, long-term memory skills, and cognitive/thinking skills

- Trivia/discussion groups: promote mental stimulation, long-term memory skills, and cognitive/thinking skills

Recommended group size: Medium to large

Suggested time frame: One hour

Special needs/ability level (physical/cognitive skills needed): All residents can take part on some level.

Activity outline:

- Share the history of Thanksgiving (use the Internet as a resource), do some Thanksgiving trivia, and discuss traditions of Thanksgiving and family gatherings

- Go around the room and ask everyone to name something for which he or she is thankful

- Serve hot apple cider and pumpkin bars

For each activity, always welcome everyone to the group and always close the activity with a "Goodbye" and "See you next time." Praise and thank everyone for their participation.

Variations/adaptations/modifications: Show a Thanksgiving slide show as part of the group.

Helpful hints/notes: Observe all infection-control guidelines and individual resident dietary needs/restrictions when serving food and beverages. Much of the setup for this event can be done prior to gathering residents so that you are ready to begin once residents have gathered. Assemble all needed equipment and supplies prior to the start of this activity.

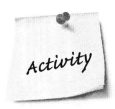

Activity

Wedding Week

Target audience: Residents who enjoy social opportunities, based on resident interests and needs

Objectives/outcomes:

- Promotes social interaction among peers, family members, and the staff

- Provides for companionship and conversation

- Promotes reminiscence, mental stimulation, long-term memory skills, and cognitive/ thinking skills

- Provides a learning opportunity

Recommended group size: Medium to large (varies based on activity)

Suggested time frame: One hour for each activity

Special needs/ability level (physical/cognitive skills needed): Primarily residents with moderate to high cognitive functioning. Ability to follow directions, complete tasks, respond verbally, and interact on some level.

Activity outline:

- Schedule a wedding display: Ask residents/families and the staff for wedding dresses, wedding pictures, and other wedding-related items for your display. Set up the display for a day that people can go through at their leisure. (Make sure everything is marked to be returned to their rightful owners.)

- Schedule a wedding cake decorating demonstration and save the cake for the "wedding reception." (The decorator may donate his or her time and cake for the free advertising.)

- Schedule a floral demonstration (silk or real flowers) and use the resultant bouquets and boutonnières for the "wedding."

- Schedule a bridal shower for the ladies. Offer mini spa treatments (e.g., facials, massages) and give the "bride" a spa basket. Play some traditional bridal shower games. Serve tea or wine and snacks.

- Schedule a bachelor party for the men. Serve beer and snacks. Invite belly dancers to come and perform (universities and dance studios sometimes have belly dancing groups).

- Plan a mock wedding. Select a bride, groom, maid of honor, best man, bridesmaids, and groomsmen. Have the women visit the beauty shop to have their hair and make-up done prior to the wedding. Have the administrator walk the bride down the aisle, and have other staff members escort the rest of the bridal party down the aisle. Have someone "officiate" the ceremony. Try to get as many staff members involved as possible; make this a facility-wide event. Perform a "real" pretend ceremony. Secure suits and dresses for the bridal party ahead of time. Have all residents "dress up" for the wedding. The week prior to the wedding, deliver wedding invitations to all residents. (You can make these on the computer.) Hold the wedding reception immediately after the mock wedding. Have a band/entertainment. Serve wedding cake and punch. Toast the bride and groom with champagne. Have them feed each other cake. Have the bride and groom have a special dance. Have the bride dance with the administrator. Take lots of pictures and then make a "wedding album" and put it out for residents and families to look through.

For each activity, always welcome everyone to the group and always close the activity with a "Goodbye" and "See you next time." Praise and thank everyone for their participation.

Variations/adaptations/modifications: Instead of a weeklong event, you can just make the "mock wedding" be funny by turning it into a mock "hillbilly wedding." Have the angry father come with a shotgun to stop the wedding when the preacher says, "If anyone feels these two should not be married, speak now or forever hold your peace." Have the staff/residents act the parts humorously. The bridal party can wear bib overalls; use your imagination. This would just be a one-day event. Instead of a wedding display, you could schedule a wedding attire fashion show and have female models wear wedding and bridesmaid dresses and male models wear suits.

Helpful hints/notes: Encourage residents' families and staff members to take part in these events. Much of the setup for these events can be done prior to gathering residents so that you are ready to begin once residents have gathered. Observe all infection-control guidelines and individual resident dietary needs/restrictions when serving food and beverages. Assemble all needed equipment and supplies prior to the start of each activity. Save all the information you've gathered for this event, laminate it or put it in plastic sleeves, and place it in a binder or folder labeled "Wedding Week," and you now have an annual event already planned for years to come.

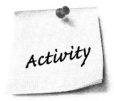

Western Day

Target audience: Residents who enjoy social opportunities, based on resident interests and needs

Objectives/outcomes:

- Promotes social interaction between peers and the staff, mental stimulation, and recreation.

- Provides for companionship, refreshments, and conversation.

- Provides a learning opportunity.

- Western roundup recreational games: provide opportunities for physical exercise and friendly competition in a recreational setting. To maintain and improve fine and gross motor skills. To maintain and improve hand-eye coordination. To develop a sense of pride and self-esteem associated with friendly competition and team play.

Recommended group size: Small or large (varies based on activity)

Suggested time frame: 30 – 60 minutes for each activity

Special needs/ability level (physical/cognitive skills needed): Primarily residents with moderate to high cognitive functioning. Ability to follow directions, complete tasks, respond verbally, and interact on some level.

Activity outline:

- Have the Dietary Department plan a Western dinner for all residents (serve BBQ or an "on the trail" roundup meal). Promote conversations with open-ended questions and encourage peer conversations. Play background country western music to set the mood (in all dining areas), and to develop a pleasant and appropriate atmosphere.

- Conduct Western roundup recreational games: Have someone bring in a saddle and a "horse" to set it on. Have residents try to lasso the saddle horn with the rope. We have standup horses for a floor horse race game that we set around the room and residents try to lasso them with the rope. You could also set up full 2-liter bottles on a table or the floor; secure rings to the rope and have residents try to lasso the bottles with the rings on the ropes. (This is easier than the aforementioned options.)

- Gunfight at the O.K. Corral: Set up some targets. These can be empty water bottles, empty cans, or some other targets that are easy to knock over. Have residents shoot at the targets using cork guns. (Keep resident safety in mind and make sure the cork guns are never aimed at anyone. Use safety glasses. Provide adequate supervision throughout the activity.) Give one point for each target a resident knocks over. Keep track of scores; the person with the highest score is the winner. (Men especially will like this activity.)

- Kitty's Saloon: Set up a saloon with a bar, use a "player piano" or Disklavier (this is a piano that plays itself, just like a player piano) if you are lucky enough to have one, play background country western music, or have a live entertainer perform country western music. Have staff members dress the part of "Kitty" the saloon owner and other saloon gals (tastefully, of course) who will serve residents drinks. Offer beer, wine, "moonshine," mixed drinks, and nonalcoholic beverages. Serve peanuts in the shell, and puffed popcorn or regular popcorn (depending on your residents' diets). Promote conversations with open-ended questions and encourage peer conversations.

- Have a "barn" dance. Set hay bales around the room to use instead of chairs, attempt to turn the activity area into a "barn" for the afternoon and decorate the area accordingly (e.g., with saddles, bridles, etc.). Secure a country western band if available, or use CDs. Encourage residents to clap, tap their toes, stomp their feet, dance, or move to the music, even if they're in wheelchairs. You could also secure square dancers to come and "kick off" the barn dance with square dance demonstrations.

- Show an old Wild West video/DVD (John Wayne is usually well received), or show old Western TV shows that are now on video/DVD (e.g., *Bonanza, Gun Smoke, Maverick, Have Gun Will Travel,* and *The Virginian*; search the Internet for popular shows of the 1950s). This activity can be done for a small or large group, or as an independent in-room activity.

For each activity, always welcome everyone to the group and always close the activity with a "Goodbye" and "See you next time." Praise and thank everyone for their participation.

Variations/adaptations/modifications: Some of the activities may be offered one-on-one with residents who are unwilling or unable to participate in a group. You will need to simplify tasks, make adaptations (they may need closer targets, or verbal and visual cues), and offer more assistance to those residents with diminished abilities (they may be able to perform tasks with direct hand-over-hand guidance). Some activities can include low-functioning residents when adaptations/modifications are made.

Helpful hints/notes: Decorate the dining and activity areas in a Western theme. Encourage residents and staff members to dress in Western attire for the day (bandanas, Western shirts, Western skirts, cowboy hats, etc.). Observe all infection-control guidelines and individual resident dietary needs/restrictions when serving food and beverages. You must know of any food allergies your residents may have. Much of the setup for the events can be done prior to gathering residents so that you are ready to begin once residents have gathered. Assemble all needed equipment and supplies prior to the start of each activity. Encourage a positive atmosphere for fair, fun recreational play and competition. Announce and congratulate winners and players. Watch for signs of any residents becoming overly tired or too competitive. Save all the information you've gathered for this event, laminate it or put it in plastic sleeves, and place it in a binder or folder labeled "Western Day," and you now have an annual event already planned for years to come.

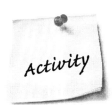

Activity

Wine and Cheese Tasting

Target audience: Residents who enjoy social opportunities, based on resident interests and needs

Objectives/outcomes:

- Promotes social interaction between peers and the staff

- Provides for companionship, refreshments, and conversation

Recommended group size: Medium to large

Suggested time frame: One hour

Special needs/ability level (physical/cognitive skills needed): Primarily residents with moderate to high cognitive functioning

Activity outline:

- Offer a variety of white, red, and blush wines (offer nonalcoholic wine as well), oyster crackers (or a variety of crackers), and a variety of cheeses cut into squares or slices for residents to taste

- Play classical background music or have a harpist if able

- Serve wine in wine glasses

Welcome everyone to the group and close the activity with a "Goodbye" and "See you next time." Praise and thank everyone for their participation.

Helpful hints/notes: Observe all infection-control guidelines and individual resident dietary needs/restrictions when serving food and beverages. Much of the setup for this event can be done prior to gathering residents so that you are ready to begin once residents have gathered. Assemble all needed equipment and supplies prior to the start of the activity.

Winter Charades

Target audience: Residents who enjoy social opportunities and acting, based on resident interests and needs

Objectives/outcomes:

- Promotes social interaction between peers and the staff

- Provides for companionship and conversation

- Promotes reminiscence, memory recall, mental stimulation, long-term memory skills, and cognitive/thinking skills

- Provides opportunities for recognition and builds self-esteem

Recommended group size: Medium

Suggested time frame: One hour

Special needs/ability level (physical/cognitive skills needed): Primarily residents with moderate to high cognitive functioning. Ability to follow directions, complete tasks, respond verbally, and interact on some level. Ability to read and act out words. Cognitive reasoning skills. Because the words often draw on long-term memory, residents with moderate cognitive impairments can do surprisingly well with charades.

Activity outline:

- Choose your winter charade words ahead of time. Print them out and laminate them. Save them in a large manila envelope.

- Place the words face down in a basket.

- Ask for a resident to volunteer to go first by picking a card. He or she then acts out the word he or she chose. The staff can help residents who cannot come up with a way to act out the word they chose, but give residents ample time to do this themselves first, and encourage them to think for themselves. The staff may also want to demonstrate how to play the game before the first resident takes his or her turn.

- Whoever guesses correctly first gets to pick the next word, and so on. If the same residents keep winning turns, you will need to let other residents have a turn before the end of the game.

For this activity, welcome everyone to the group and close the activity with a "Goodbye" and "See you next time." Praise and thank everyone for their participation.

Variations/adaptations/modifications: Residents can come up with their own words based on other topics for charades based on different themes.

Helpful hints/notes: Much of the setup for this event can be done prior to gathering residents so that you are ready to begin once residents have gathered. Assemble all needed equipment and supplies prior to the start of the activity.

Winter Olympics Week

Target audience: Residents who enjoy social opportunities and friendly competition, based on resident interests and needs

Objectives/outcomes:

- Promotes social interaction among peers, family members, and the staff.

- Provides for companionship and conversation.

- Promotes reminiscence, mental stimulation, long-term memory skills, and cognitive/thinking skills.

- Provides a learning opportunity.

- Provides an opportunity for recognition.

- Provides opportunities for physical exercise and friendly competition in a recreational setting. To maintain and improve fine and gross motor skills. To maintain and improve hand-eye coordination. To develop a sense of pride and self-esteem associated with friendly competition and team play.

Recommended group size: Medium to large (varies based on activity)

Suggested time frame: 30 – 60 minutes for each activity

Special needs/ability level (physical/cognitive skills needed): Primarily residents with moderate to high cognitive functioning. Ability to follow directions, complete tasks, respond verbally, and interact on some level.

Activity outline:

- This is a great activity to do in coordination with the real Winter Olympics every four years (but you can do it annually). It gives residents something to look forward to following the holidays, which can be a letdown.

- Purchase gold, silver, and bronze medals from a party supply store or catalog. Use the file labeled Winter Olympics located on your CD-ROM for your opening ceremony.

- Plan your weeklong events. Aim to have two events daily: one in the morning and one in the afternoon. Complete the Olympic Competitor's Registration Sheet the week prior to the event located on the CD-ROM. Advertise your event several weeks prior with a poster located on the CD-ROM and a banner or flag with the Olympic rings on it (you can make one out of cloth and fabric paint as part of a group project with the residents).

- The first event is the opening ceremony. You can purchase a battery-operated flashlight torch for a resident to carry. Have a torch relay from one unit to the next prior to your opening ceremony. Have all residents then gather in the activity area for the official opening ceremony. Have the Resident Council president declare the official beginning of the Winter Olympics by saying, "Let the Games begin." Use an outdoor Christmas plug-in candle that is 2 – 3 feet tall, and have it represent the torch that is lit during the opening ceremony and that remains lit until the closing ceremony. (Cover the bottom of the candle with black poster board and make a funnel shape at the top. Leave only the "wick" of the candle showing.)

- Schedule daily competitive events (e.g., bowling, ring toss, golf putting, snowball throwing [use Styrofoam craft balls and ice cream buckets, six in a row, getting progressively farther away], target darts, basketball, a trivia rally competition, or other competitive recreational games of interest to your residents). Use the Olympic score sheets to keep track of the gold, silver, and bronze winners. These are located on the CD-ROM.

- Hold the closing ceremony as the last event. Have all residents gathered in the activity area for the official closing ceremony. Residents' family members can attend as well. The activities director can be the spokesperson/announcer for the awards, but have the administrator hand out the awards. (Put the medal around the winner's neck and kiss him or her on the cheek.) Also hand out Certificates of Merit (made out ahead of time for each resident who participated in the Games; a sample is available located on the CD-ROM. In addition, hand out Certificates of Merit in such categories as Good Sportsmanship, Most Determined, Best Effort, Most Motivated, and Best Cheerleader, made out ahead of time, for those participants who did not receive a gold, silver, or bronze medal; a sample is available located on the CD-ROM. This way, every participant leaves the event with two forms of recognition. Have enough volunteers on hand to bring residents to the front of the room to receive their medals and have their pictures taken.

- Encourage participants to display their paper certificates on their doors or in their rooms and to wear their medals for a week or two, which will encourage others to ask them what they got the award for, thereby making this a constant reinforcement of a significant achievement and source of pride. (Residents take so much pride in this that they have been buried with their certificates and medals.)

Welcome everyone to the group and close the activity with a "Goodbye" and "See you next time." Praise and thank everyone for their participation.

Variations/adaptations/modifications: You will need to simplify tasks, make adaptations (certain residents may need closer targets, or verbal and visual cues), and offer more assistance to those residents with diminished abilities (they may be able to perform tasks with direct hand-over-hand guidance). Some activities can include low-functioning residents when adaptations/modifications are made.

Helpful hints/notes: Much of the setup for this event can be done prior to gathering residents so that you are ready to begin once residents have gathered. Assemble all needed equipment and supplies prior to the start of the activity. Encourage a positive atmosphere for fair, fun recreational play and competition. Save all the information you've gathered for this event, laminate it or put it in plastic sleeves, and place it in a binder or folder labeled "Winter Olympics Week," and you now have an annual event already planned for years to come.

Chapter 4

Activities for Residents with Dementia, Alzheimer's, and Behavioral Issues

Considerable research documents the health benefits of remaining active as you age and the importance of remaining engaged in meaningful activities. Providing meaningful and engaging activities to residents with dementia and those who exhibit behavioral symptoms is extremely important. Activity interventions can help residents to maintain their remaining abilities for a longer period of time, can provide stimulation, solace, comfort, and relaxation, and can help to eliminate symptomatic behaviors.

In 2006, the Centers for Medicare & Medicaid Services issued new guidance for activities that specifically directed facilities to improve activities for residents with Alzheimer's disease and other forms of dementia. The expectation is that facilities will provide all residents, even those with advanced dementia, with individualized, "person-centered" activities. Your facility's policy should be to offer supportive programs to residents with varying stages of impaired cognition and perceptual abilities. These supportive programs promote resident awareness, responsiveness, and participation that are consistent with individual interests, needs, and ability levels.

Stages of Dementia

There are different stages or levels of dementia, with each stage reflecting progressive declines in cognition and physical abilities. In this book, we will refer to these stages as *mild*, *moderate*, and *severe*. Each stage of dementia impacts a resident's cognitive function, which includes language, processing speed, hand-eye coordination, verbal memory, learning ability, visual memory, and the ability to plan and carry out tasks.

Symptoms of a person suffering from *mild dementia* are mild forgetfulness (memory loss of recent events), and mild impairments in language (difficulty finding the right words), abstract thinking, attention span, decision-making, orientation (altered concept of time), ability to concentrate, memory recall, and ability to learn new things. At this stage, people suffering from mild dementia are often aware of their memory loss and can be embarrassed by it and attempt to hide it, often using humor. (Generally, these people can still do these things, but it takes them a longer period of time and they may require cueing to aid in their memory process.)

People suffering from *moderate dementia* exhibit increased deterioration in cognitive functioning (their symptoms become more obvious), increased disorientation/profound memory loss (they may confuse the past with the present and "live" in the past; i.e., their children become their sisters and brothers, etc.), decreased language abilities (they may start to mix nonsensical words with real words and have garbled speech, repetitive speech, word-finding difficulty, perseverate speech, and/or difficulty naming objects or maintaining a logical conversation), loss of safety awareness resulting in an increase in falls, and the need for reminders, redirection, verbal and visual cues, and direct physical guidance to complete tasks. At this stage, you may see changes in the resident's mood and behavior: for example, yelling or calling out, shadowing others/not wanting to be alone, wandering, withdrawal, anxiety, depression, agitation, aggression, paranoia, and changes in sleeping patterns.

People suffering from *severe dementia* exhibit a lack of name and face recognition, are nonverbal or just make vocal noises, have difficulty swallowing/eating, and may keep their eyes closed much of the time. They have forgotten basic skills, may lose weight, have decreased physical movement, and respond only minimally to stimuli and their environment (they may be devoid of affect and awareness).

It is important to remember that the attention span of a memory-impaired resident can be as short as two minutes or as long as 45 minutes, depending on the type of activity being offered (a more engaging activity usually increases a resident's attention span). In addition, the environment can affect a resident's attention span. For instance, an overstimulating environment can cause increased anxiety and agitation, therefore limiting the resident's attention span.

Additional factors that can affect a resident's attention span include environmental distractions (you should limit distractions as much as possible), the time of day (each resident has his or her own biological clock which can determine certain times of the day as being better than others for activity participation), and the resident's health status (e.g., fatigue, illness). The resident's mood also can affect his or her attention span (i.e., the resident has to be in the right frame of mind to participate in an activity).

Activities for residents with dementia

Activities for residents in the mild and moderate stages of dementia should focus on maintaining or improving the residents' functional and cognitive abilities. You can achieve this by providing a routine, adapting programs for safety, modifying activities, providing verbal and visual cues and direct physical guidance and prompts, being flexible in your approach, optimizing the resident's sense of success, modifying the environment and routine, preserving function, minimizing agitation, and validating what the resident is saying. Activities for residents in the severe stage of dementia should focus on providing stimulation, comfort, solace, and relaxation, as you will not be able to improve their functional and cognitive abilities. (Activities for residents in the mild and moderate stages should also focus on providing these benefits if the facility has determined that they would benefit such residents.) For residents with very limited responses/abilities, offer environmental and sensory stimulation while taking into account their interests and needs. You can achieve this by providing constant direction and supervision, accommodating wandering, building on any retained abilities no matter how small, and providing comfort care.

Communicating with residents with dementia

Communicating with residents with dementia provides its own unique challenges. Keep these general principles in mind:

- Approach the resident calmly and cheerfully in an adult fashion

- Correct any hearing or visual problems

- Remove distractions

- Avoid overwhelming the resident physically or verbally

- Presume comprehension on some level and remember non-verbal communication becomes more important as the disease progresses

Some key points for verbal communication include:

- Using concrete phrases

- Speaking slowly and distinctly

- Asking one question at a time and waiting for a response

- Offering simple choices

- Providing praise and reassurance

- Validating feelings

- Using the KISS method: Keep it Short and Simple

Some key points for non-verbal communication include:

- Remembering that residents can pick up on your attitude and mood

- Watching for their non-verbal messages as a clue to problems

- Using non-threatening postures and gestures

- Demonstrating desired actions

- Conveying a positive/supportive attitude

- Standing or sitting at their level

- Moving slowly

- Using touch and allowing them to touch you/hold your hand

- Gently stroking

- Putting your arm around their shoulder (always assess what they are comfortable with in regard to touch)

- Encouraging communication via nods, smiles, and eye contact

- Trying to understand the feelings behind their confusing words

Behaviors are a form of communication, a symptom of an unmet need. They are not a form of acting out or seeking attention. The behavior is not challenging for the resident (though it certainly can be distressing to him or her); often the resident is communicating in the only way he or she knows because of his or her cognitive impairments. The challenge is for the staff to figure out why the resident is exhibiting a certain behavior, developing effective individualized interventions, discovering the antecedents to the behavior, and putting measures in place (a care plan) to ward off future behaviors. Activity interventions can play a huge role in reducing and eliminating behaviors. All staff members can and should utilize activity interventions (the activities staff usually is not available 24/7).

Specialized Dementia Programming and Multisensory Rooms

Many facilities typically do not provide enough low-functioning programs on a daily basis, which can lead to deficiencies in their programs as a whole. A multisensory room provides a place for residents to go that is stress-free and stimulating. Specialized dementia programming provides group activities in an environment that is success-oriented, failure-free, purposeful, engaging, and meaningful. Such programs can help you with appropriate programming and positive survey outcomes. Surveyors like to see multisensory rooms in which specific dementia programming is occurring, as it means you have great programs for low-functioning residents, which could result in a deficiency-free survey.

These programs offer many benefits, including the following:

- Residents are aware of the comfort and enjoyment they receive from these programs

- The programs become a part of residents' daily routines and residents recognize you and their peers

- The strong relationships residents naturally build via these programs create a "family" feel to the unit/program

- Residents warmly welcome you and "come along" with you eagerly as they feel more connected to each other

- Residents have a more enriched lifestyle, and are calmer, more content, happier, and joyful in their expressions

- Agitation and negative behaviors (restlessness, anxiety) decrease and residents are more relaxed

- You are able to reach residents with whom it has been difficult to establish contact

- Residents become more responsive and participative

- The familiarity with day-to-day experiences helps to establish security, trust, and comfort, thereby increasing residents' social opportunities

- The consistency that is provided via these groups enables meaningful activity experiences with positive outcomes

- Residents become more in tune to what is going on in their environment

- Success and active engagement in each activity are a direct result of the activity being specifically geared to each resident's ability level, both physical and cognitive

- Residents become more animated, talkative, and humorous

- Residents are less apathetic, show more emotion, and behave in a "normal" social way because you are recognizing them for who they are and where they are, and you are helping them to remember their strengths and importance, rather than reminding them of all that they have lost

- Medication can be significantly reduced for these residents because of the positive changes the programming and environment make in their daily lives

Typical activity programs place pressure on residents to perform, which for dementia residents leads to anxiety, agitation, and frustration. A multisensory room introduces pleasurable experiences that provide residents with the opportunity to attain happiness and purpose, and to improve their quality of life without any rules or expectations of performance, so they maintain control. These programs also actively engage residents in activities that gently stimulate their senses throughout the day, so residents are not just sitting in chairs doing nothing and with no interaction provided. Being active and engaged is a key component of these programs; without this, you do not achieve positive outcomes.

Multisensory rooms provide unique benefits for a variety of populations, including those with special needs, dementia, and chronic pain. The following types of residents should be included in multisensory room and small-group dementia-specific programs:

- Individuals with dementia/cognitive impairment

- Those who display repetitive, self-stimulating actions (rubbing, picking)

- Those with limited or absent verbal skills

- Those who do not benefit from a group setting

- Those who show patterns of agitation and anxious behaviors

- Those with limited responses or who are nonresponsive

- Individuals with chronic pain issues

A multisensory room is effective for individual, one-on-one, or small-group participation. Remember, the focus with specialized dementia programming is to provide more one-on-one attention so that these residents are more actively engaged. Therefore, you must keep in mind your staff-to-resident ratio. For specialized small-group programming, the recommended time is generally 30 minutes, with some variation based on the resident's response and attention span. However, the recommended time could be as short as 20 minutes or as long as 45 minutes; use as your guide the engagement level of those who are participating. You may move on to another group once an activity is complete, or if residents are no longer engaged in the activity. Session length for a multisensory room program or experience can be as short as 10 minutes, depending on the person's attention span. Various sensorial materials should be available. (See the Multisensory Room Policy and Procedure for examples.)

Your facility's multisensory room should be available 24/7 for dementia resident use. It is expected that all staff members who work on the unit will utilize the room with residents, and staff members are strongly encouraged to do so when properly oriented to the use of the room. Proper training of all staff members who work on the unit is necessary so that everyone knows the benefits of involving residents in its use and how to conduct activities that are beneficial to each specific resident.

A multisensory room is most effective if it is used prior to a resident becoming significantly agitated. The environment can have the opposite effect if a resident is allowed to reach a severely agitated state, and the resident's behavior may worsen if the environment is overstimulating. It's important to note that residents may find certain things within the room frightening or upsetting; hence, documentation of resident responses, both positive and negative, is crucial to creating the best environment for each resident. Approaches that are most effective for an individual should be repeated and those that have a negative impact should not be repeated. For this reason, each use of the multisensory room should be by a group of residents with similar needs and preferences. Never assume that if a resident has a negative response to the room that he or she will never have a positive response, because the mood of a person with dementia can change by the moment. Multisensory rooms are for enjoyable, failure-free experiences with no expectation of performance.

Include some or all of the following programs for your residents with dementia to provide them with stimulating, comforting, meaningful, and engaging activities.

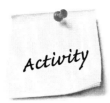

Activity

ABC Game

Target audience: Residents needing specialized dementia programming

Objectives/outcomes:

- To provide visual stimulation and increase responsiveness

- To provide an opportunity for simple communication

- To promote communication and enjoyment

- To encourage interaction with others and increase social contact

- To enhance/increase attention span and memory recall, thinking and reasoning skills, concentration, and identification of letters and words

- To promote the ability to follow one-step directions

- To improve mood by actively engaging residents at their level of ability

Recommended group size: Small

Suggested time frame: 30 – 45 minutes

Special needs/ability level (physical/cognitive skills needed): Residents with the cognitive capacity to identify letters and words and to follow one-step directions. Residents with varying levels of cognitive/physical abilities can join this group, as you work with them individually and provide needed assistance at their ability level. You need to make sure that residents are able to achieve some level of success in this activity for it to be beneficial to them.

Activity outline:

- You will need cards with the letters of the alphabet on them. It is also helpful to have pictures of words that begin with each letter of the alphabet and cards with the words spelled out.

- Start by showing a card with one letter of the alphabet. Ask the resident to identify the letter. Then ask if he or she can think of a word that begins with that letter, and show the resident a picture (if you are using pictures) of an object that begins with that letter. Lastly, show the resident a card with the word representing the object in the picture (if you are using word and picture cards) and ask him or her to read it. Residents can be very cognitively impaired but still be able to read, so even if they cannot think of a word that begins with a certain letter, they can read the word and then you can ask them whether that word begins with that letter. This is why it's nice to have all three types of cards. It will allow most residents to have some measure of success at their ability level. As you go through the different letters, initiate a discussion about the words on the cards. You will not get through the entire alphabet in one session, which would be overwhelming for dementia residents. The next time you play the game, use different letters of the alphabet.

- Work with each resident individually as needed, but let each resident do as much as he or she is capable and provide assistance only if it is truly needed (e.g., you may need to point out a card, but the resident may be able to turn it over him or herself).

- You can also use an aromatherapy diffuser with a scent that promotes mental stimulation, such as citrus or peppermint.

Variations/adaptations/modifications: You have to adapt/modify your approach based on the cognitive ability level of each individual within the group. Go around and provide the visual, verbal, and direct physical guidance that each person needs to be successful. Redirect as necessary. You will need to offer more assistance to residents with diminished abilities. This requires that you have assessed the abilities and identified the needs, interests, and interventions of each resident in attendance. A variation of this activity is to give residents a category (e.g., name two fruits that begin with the letter A, name two sports that begin with the letter B, name three desserts that begin with the letter C, etc.). You should keep the list to five at most. Another variation is to pick a topic (e.g., animals) and then have residents name as many words as they can that begin with each letter of the alphabet within that topic; you can write the words on a whiteboard so that the residents can see how many they came up with, and to serve as a visual reminder and aid in memory recall.

Helpful hints/notes: You can purchase cards for this program or make them yourself. To make your own cards use a computer and clipart, type the words in a large, easy-to-read, boldface font, print them on card stock, laminate them, and use a paper cutter to cut them out. This will be time-consuming, but if you have a limited budget or cannot find these cards in a store (even a school supply store) you will still be able to conduct this effective dementia program with your residents. Utilize student volunteers to save time. Many high schools require students to do volunteer hours, and some Girl Scout troops may be interested in helping out as a way to earn Girl Scout badges. Much of the setup for this activity can be done prior to gathering residents so that you are ready to begin once residents have gathered. Assemble all needed equipment and supplies prior to the start of the activity.

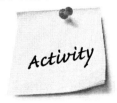

Afternoon Multisensory Room Program

Target audience: Residents needing specialized dementia programming and those with behavior issues

Objectives/outcomes:

- To provide tactile, auditory, olfactory, and visual stimulation and increase responsiveness

- To provide an opportunity for simple communication

- To promote relaxation, solace, pain management, and enjoyment

- To encourage interaction with others and increase social contact

- To decrease the frequency and severity of symptomatic behavior (tension, anxiety, and agitation)

- To stimulate the senses of withdrawn residents

- To soothe/relax residents who are agitated

- To improve relationships between caregivers and residents

Recommended group size: Small group, interacting one-on-one

Suggested time frame: Approximately five minutes per resident

Special needs/ability level (physical/cognitive skills needed): Residents with varying levels of cognitive/physical abilities can join this group, as you work with them individually and provide needed assistance at their ability level. You need to make sure residents are able to achieve some level of success in this activity for it to be beneficial to them.

Activity outline:

- After lunch, bring the residents into the multisensory room. If you do not have such a room at your facility, make the room as relaxing as possible with subdued lighting and minimal outside distractions. Place residents in a circle around the room.

- Have soft, relaxing background music playing as they gather. This creates a calming, enveloping mood.

- Greet each resident by name and with a gentle touch or hug. Make sure residents are comfortable, which may mean placing them in more comfortable chairs than wheelchairs.

- Play a nature video such as one with rainforest scenes, as this is relaxing and soothing after lunch when many residents are tired after the physical exertion of eating. The splashes of color and the movement of waterfalls or animals also seem to attract the attention of some residents, as do movies showing children and animals in action, and old television shows and movies. You can also use videos of fish, flowers, and the ocean.

- You want to create a restful environment so that participants do not notice the distraction of "change of shift."

- Use the multisensory room equipment to provide relaxation and stimulation (moving lights, lava lamps, waterfalls, bubble walls, bead curtains, etc.). Use a variety of items for participants to explore their surroundings. This can include pinwheels, colorful small balls, stuffed animals, and other tactile objects that residents can manipulate with repetitive motions.

- Engage participants in passive range of motion (ROM) activities/exercises to include slow movement of the hands, fingers, arms, feet, and legs. Play some upbeat music for this portion of the activity.

- You may want to offer residents the opportunity to soak their feet in warm water, and then gently massaging their feet with lotion. This is a very basic and loving experience and complete bliss for many participants. (Make sure there are no contraindications for this.)

- Offer residents a treat in the afternoon that is within their dietary guidelines (e.g., lollipop, ice cream, pudding, yogurt, etc.).

- Provide residents with supportive RO while working with them (talk about the weather, the present season, upcoming holidays, current happenings in the nursing home, their family, etc.).

- You can also use an aromatherapy diffuser with a scent that promotes relaxation, such as vanilla or lavender, or a seasonal scent (e.g., spices or cinnamon for winter; rain, or lily of the valley, lilacs, or hyacinths for spring; watermelon or roses for summer; and pumpkin or apples and cinnamon for fall).

Variations/adaptations/modifications: You have to adapt/modify your approach based on the physical and cognitive ability level of each individual within the group. Go around and provide the visual, verbal, and direct physical guidance that each person needs to be successful. Redirect as necessary. You will need to simplify tasks and offer more assistance to residents with diminished abilities (they may be able to perform tasks with direct hand-over-hand guidance).

Helpful hints/notes: Observe all infection-control guidelines. Much of the setup for this activity can be done prior to gathering residents so that you are ready to begin once residents have gathered. Assemble all needed equipment and supplies prior to the start of the activity. Clean and disinfect the activity supplies as needed/according to your facility's policy and procedure.

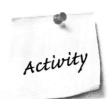
Activity

Big Ball Fun

Target audience: Residents needing specialized dementia programming and those with behavioral issues

Objectives/outcomes:

- To provide visual and tactile stimulation and increase responsiveness

- To provide an opportunity for simple communication

- To provide a pleasurable, failure-free, and stress-free environment

- To allow individuals the time, space, and opportunity to enjoy the environment at their own pace, free from unrealistic expectations of others

- To promote large motor physical activity and lower body range of motion, communication, and enjoyment

- To encourage interaction with others and increase social contact

- To enhance/increase attention span and concentration and promote the ability to follow one-step directions or mimic desired actions

- To improve mood by actively engaging residents at their level of ability

- To provide an atmosphere that encourages participants to explore their environment and to be able to enjoy themselves

- To promote the ability for residents to express themselves

- To promote person-centered care

- To improve relationships between caregivers and residents

Recommended group size: Medium

Suggested time frame: 30 – 45 minutes

Special needs/ability level (physical/cognitive skills needed): Residents with the physical capacity to kick a ball, follow one-step directions, or mimic desired actions. You need to make sure that residents are able to achieve some level of success in this activity for it to be beneficial to them.

Activity outline:

- You will need a large, brightly colored ball (the ones physical therapy uses and that are used for Pilates/exercises). They are available from sporting goods companies.

- Play some background music that will promote physical activity (ragtime, marching bands, etc.).

- Have residents sit in a large circle and kick the ball back and forth.

- If they have foot pedals and they are able, take their feet off the pedals and turn the pedals to the sides so that the residents can kick the ball when it comes to them.

- You can also use an aromatherapy diffuser with a scent that promotes physical activity and mental stimulation, such as citrus or peppermint.

Variations/adaptations/modifications: You have to adapt/modify your approach based on the physical and cognitive ability level of each individual within the group. Go around and provide the visual, verbal, and direct physical guidance that each person needs to be successful. Redirect as necessary. You will need to offer more assistance to residents with diminished abilities (they may be able to perform tasks with direct hand-over-hand guidance). This requires that you have assessed the abilities and identified the needs, interests, and interventions of each resident in attendance. As a variation, you can turn this into a dodge ball game with a staff member in the center. You can also utilize a medium-size, soft ball or beach ball and have the residents toss the ball and then catch it to get some upper-body range of motion as well and to extend or break up the activity.

Helpful hints/notes: Much of the setup for this activity can be done prior to gathering residents so that you are ready to begin once residents have gathered. Assemble all needed equipment and supplies prior to the start of the activity. Clean and disinfect the activity supplies as needed/according to your facility's policy and procedure.

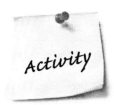
Activity

Bubble Mania

Target audience: Residents needing specialized dementia programming and those with behavior issues

Objectives/outcomes:

- To provide visual and tactile stimulation and increase responsiveness

- To provide an opportunity for simple communication

- To promote communication and enjoyment

- To encourage interaction with others and increase social contact

- To enhance/increase attention span, promote physical movement, and improve/ encourage range of motion and free-form movement

- To promote relaxation

- To decrease the frequency and severity of symptomatic behavior (tension, anxiety, and agitation)

- To stimulate the senses of withdrawn residents

- To soothe/relax residents who are agitated

- To improve relationships between caregivers and residents

- To improve mood by actively engaging residents at their level of ability

Recommended group size: Small

Suggested time frame: 30 minutes

Special needs/ability level (physical/cognitive skills needed): Residents with varying levels of cognitive/physical abilities can join this group, as you work with them individually and provide needed assistance at their ability level. You need to make sure that residents are able to achieve some level of success in this activity for it to be beneficial to them.

Activity outline:

- You will need a bubble machine. Place a bath towel or a blanket on the floor to catch the bubbles as the soap mixture can make the floor very slippery.

- Set up the bubble machine and place the residents in a semicircle around the machine, but within reach of the bubbles.

- At first, just ask them to look at the bubbles and notice the different sizes. Do not provide instructions initially, so you can see the types of reactions the residents exhibit on their own. Most likely, they will start to reach for the bubbles, trying to catch them and pop them without any prompting. Eventually, prompt residents with verbal cues who do not react on their own. This is great range of motion exercise. Allow the activity to continue for as long as it holds the interest of the majority of the residents. Prompt residents for discussion by asking simple, direct questions (e.g., do you remember popping bubbles when you were small? What do bubbles remind you of? Did you ever take bubble baths?).

- You can also use an aromatherapy diffuser with a scent that promotes relaxation, such as vanilla or lavender. Bubbles naturally are soothing. Breaking the bubbles helps to eliminate aggression/agitation for some residents.

- You may play background music that promotes relaxation (e.g., classical or Lawrence Welk music).

Variations/adaptations/modifications: You could follow this activity with a Lawrence Welk video/DVD when residents lose interest in the bubbles.

Helpful hints/notes: Much of the setup for this activity can be done prior to gathering residents so that you are ready to begin once residents have gathered. Assemble all needed equipment and supplies prior to the start of the activity.

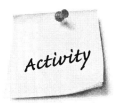

Activity **Colors and Shapes Bingo**

Target audience: Residents needing specialized dementia programming

Objectives/outcomes:

- To provide visual stimulation and increase responsiveness

- To provide an opportunity for simple communication

- To promote communication and enjoyment

- To encourage interaction with others and increase social contact

- To enhance/increase attention span and memory recall, thinking and reasoning skills, concentration, and identification of colors and shapes, and promote ability to follow one-step directions

- To improve mood by actively engaging residents at their level of ability

Recommended group size: Small

Suggested time frame: 30 – 45 minutes

Special needs/ability level (physical/cognitive skills needed): Residents with the cognitive capacity to identify colors and shapes. Residents with varying levels of cognitive/physical abilities can join this group, as you work with them individually and provide needed assistance at their ability level. You need to make sure that residents are able to achieve some level of success in each activity for it to be beneficial to them.

Activity outline:

- You will need colors and shapes bingo cards (only nine squares, with three rows of three). You will need master cards of the colors and shapes for holding up for residents to see. Play as you would play a normal bingo game.

- Hold up one master card to provide a visual cue, and state the color and shape for the verbal cue. Repeat as needed.

- Work with each resident individually as needed, but have them do for themselves as much as they can and provide assistance only when it is truly needed (you may need to point out a color and shape, but they may be able to cover it themselves).

- You can also use an aromatherapy diffuser with a scent that promotes mental stimulation, such as citrus or peppermint.

Variations/adaptations/modifications: You have to adapt/modify your approach based on the cognitive ability level of each individual within the group. Go around and provide the visual, verbal, and direct physical guidance that each person needs to be successful. Redirect as necessary. You will need to offer more assistance to residents with diminished abilities. This requires that you have assessed the abilities and identified the needs, interests, and interventions of each resident in attendance. As variations, you can play alphabet bingo, number bingo, music bingo, sounds bingo, and simple themed or holiday bingo.

Helpful hints/notes: You can buy bingo cards (through an activity or school supply catalog) or make them yourself with card stock and laminate them. This will be time-consuming, but if you have a limited budget or cannot find the cards premade, making them yourself will enable you to conduct this effective dementia program with your residents. Utilize student volunteers to save yourself some time. Many high schools require students to do volunteer hours, and some Girl Scout troops may be interested in helping out as a way to earn Girl Scout badges. Much of the setup for this activity can be done prior to gathering residents so that you are ready to begin once residents have gathered. Assemble all needed equipment and supplies prior to the start of the activity.

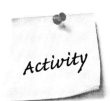

Activity | **Creative-Expressive**

Target audience: Medium- to high-functioning residents. Low-functioning with adaptations as needed and based on assessed interests and needs.

Objectives/outcomes:

- To provide creative and expressive activities for interested residents

- To allow residents to express their creative ideas

- To promote residents' positive self-esteem through participation in successful projects

- To maintain and develop fine motor skills and hand-eye coordination

- To provide residents with opportunities to express choice and preference with regard to the finished product

- To allow time for mental stimulation, peer socialization, and recreation

Recommended group size: One-on-one, small

Suggested time frame: Flexible; can range from a 15-minute visit to a 45-minute session

Activity outline:

- Equipment/materials needed: pens, pencils, paper, tape, paint, brushes, scissors* (adapted), markers, flowers, vases, yarn, baskets, glue, C-clamps, cleaning cloths, art books, and other slide/movie projector/program-specific material

- Plan your craft or topic. Prepare all materials ahead of time.

- Create an example (especially for crafts) to display to participants.

- Have all materials organized and in easily accessible containers, bags, or areas (i.e., distribute first-step materials, if appropriate).

- Display the desired outcome. Direct residents throughout the program. Provide choices.

- Seat residents around tables (round, or square for maximum assistance). Leave spaces open next to residents to permit comfortable assistance by staff members and volunteers. Introduce residents to each other. Pair up compatible residents to assist each other (e.g., two hemiplegic residents).

- Soft instrumental music may be played in the background. This generates a quiet, calm atmosphere.

- Observe the room ahead of time for good lighting, few outside distractions, comfortable temperature, and so on.

- Praise and thank residents for their participation.

- Title the artwork, identify the artist, and display the artwork as desired.

Variations/adaptations/modifications: *Use adapted materials where required; for example, to hold items securely you can use tape or clamps. Sponge-wrap pens or paint brushes for ease in handling by those with arthritic hands.

Helpful hints/notes: Take all safety precautions when conducting this activity and using these materials.

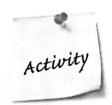 **Activity**

Creative Writing Group

Target audience: Residents with cognitive impairments (mild to moderate)

Objectives/outcomes:

- To provide visual stimulation and increase responsiveness

- To provide an opportunity for simple communication and reminiscence

- To promote communication and enjoyment

- To encourage interaction with others and increase social contact

- To enhance/increase attention span, thinking and reasoning skills, concentration, and memory recall

- To allow residents to express their creative ideas

- Promotes residents' self-esteem through successful projects

- To improve mood by actively engaging residents at their level of ability

Recommended group size: Small (8 – 12)

Suggested time frame: 30 minutes

Special needs/ability level (physical/cognitive skills needed): Residents with varying levels of cognitive/physical abilities can join this group, as you work with them individually and provide needed assistance at their ability level. They should have some remaining long-term memory skills and be able to verbally respond to simple, direct questions. You need to make sure that residents are able to achieve some level of success in this activity for it to be beneficial to them.

Activity outline:

- Greet the group and welcome each participant.

- Choose a full-page (8.5-by-11-inch) black-and-white picture and make copies so that each participant has one to look at. Crazy pictures prompt some very interesting stories. You can use pictures from magazines, newspapers, or the Internet.

- Explain in simple terms what you are going to do. For example, "I want you to look at this picture. We will talk about what you see and I will write down what you say. We will have a story at the end."

- Use a whiteboard and write down all resident responses regardless of how much sense they make to you; this is so residents have a visual of what has been said (reading is one of the last skills to go). You will also need paper and a pen to transfer residents' thoughts at the conclusion of the activity, or have another staff member or volunteer record the thoughts on paper.

- Use simple, open-ended questions to prompt verbal responses. Use who, what, where, when, and why questions. Avoid leading questions. Sample questions include: What do you see? What are they doing? Where are they? What do you think is happening? Who are they? Why do you think . . . ? Residents' answers should prompt additional questions. Once you get no more responses, the writing is complete.

- Ask residents to provide a title. If you receive no response, suggest a title.

- List all the participants as the writers, even if they did not respond verbally but were listening, as they were a part of the group.

- Collect the pictures; tell them you will return the pictures, along with the completed story, to the residents so that they can share it with their family.

- Type up the story using a large, boldface font, make copies for the residents, and pass them out along with the picture. Place the original in a book titled "Creative Resident Writings of the [facility name] Memory Care Unit," along with a copy of the picture.

Variations/adaptations/modifications: You have to adapt/modify your approach based on the physical and cognitive ability level of each individual within the group. Go around and provide the visual, verbal, and direct physical guidance that each person needs to be successful. Redirect as necessary. You will need to offer more assistance to residents with diminished abilities. This requires that you have assessed the abilities and identified the needs, interests, and interventions of each resident in attendance.

Helpful hints/notes: Much of the setup for this activity can be done prior to gathering residents so that you are ready to begin once residents have gathered. Assemble all needed equipment and supplies prior to the start of the activity.

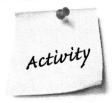

Dice Game

Target audience: Residents needing specialized dementia programming and those with behavior issues

Objectives/outcomes:

- To provide visual and tactile stimulation and increase responsiveness

- To provide an opportunity for simple communication

- To promote communication and enjoyment

- To encourage interaction with others and increase social contact

- To enhance/increase attention span and memory recall, thinking, reasoning and concentration skills, number identification, and matching skills

- To decrease the frequency and severity of symptomatic behavior (tension, anxiety, and agitation)

- To stimulate the senses of withdrawn residents

- To improve mood by actively engaging residents at their level of ability

Recommended group size: Small or one-on-one

Suggested time frame: 30 minutes

Special needs/ability level (physical/cognitive skills needed): Residents with varying levels of cognitive/physical abilities can join this group, as you work with them individually and provide needed assistance at their ability level. Residents need to be able to identify numbers on a pair of dice and be able to match them to their cards. You need to make sure that residents are able to achieve some level of success in this activity for it to be beneficial to them.

Activity outline:

- You will need cards marked with the numbers 1 through 12 (four rows of three numbers, or three rows of four numbers). Make these cards on card stock and laminate them. You will also need a pair of dice and some poker chips (or some other markers with which to cover the numbers on the cards).

- Have a resident roll the dice, then find the number of the total of the two dice (e.g., if the resident rolls a 3 and a 4, he or she would have to cover the 7 with the poker chip/marker). As an alternative, the resident can cover the 3 and the 4. Each resident takes a turn rolling the dice, and the first person to cover all of his or her numbers wins. As the game progresses, residents will not be able to cover any numbers on some rolls because they will have already covered them. This is a dice game bingo. You can award prizes, though it is not necessary as you are working on number and simple addition skills and matching skills.

- Work with each resident individually as needed, but let residents do for themselves as much as they can and provide assistance only when it is truly needed (you may need to point out a number or help them to add, but they may be able to cover the numbers themselves).

- You can also use an aromatherapy diffuser with a scent that promotes thinking and concentration, such as citrus or peppermint.

Variations/adaptations/modifications: You have to adapt/modify your approach based on the cognitive ability level of each individual. Provide the visual, verbal, and direct physical guidance that each person needs to be successful. Redirect as necessary. You will need to offer more assistance to residents with diminished abilities. This requires that you have assessed the abilities and identified the needs, interests, and interventions of each resident in attendance.

Helpful hints/notes: Utilize student volunteers to make the cards to save time. Many high schools require students to do volunteer hours, and some Girl Scout troops may be interested in helping out as a way to earn Girl Scout badges. Much of the setup for this activity can be done prior to gathering residents so that you are ready to begin once residents have gathered. Assemble all needed equipment and supplies prior to the start of the activity.

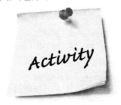

Dusterball

Target audience: Residents needing specialized dementia programming and those with behavior issues

Objectives/outcomes:

- To provide visual and tactile stimulation and increase responsiveness

- To provide an opportunity for simple communication

- To promote communication and enjoyment

- To encourage interaction with others and increase social contact

- To enhance/increase attention span and promote physical movement/large motor skills and range of motion

- To decrease the frequency and severity of symptomatic behavior (tension, anxiety, and agitation)

- To stimulate the senses of withdrawn residents

- To improve mood by actively engaging residents at their level of ability

Recommended group size: Small; enough to fit around a table

Suggested time frame: 30 minutes

Special needs/ability level (physical/cognitive skills needed): Residents with varying levels of cognitive/physical abilities can join this group, as you work with them individually and provide needed assistance at their ability level. They will need to be able to hold on to the duster with one hand. You need to make sure that residents are able to achieve some level of success in this activity for it to be beneficial to them.

Activity outline:

- You will need a small foam ball and feather or soft dusters (from four to eight, depending on the size of the table).

- Set residents up around the table (on the sides and the ends). Have them grasp the duster in one hand.

- Place the ball on the table.

- Tell them to bat the ball back and forth with the duster, trying to keep the ball on the table.

- Play lively music in the background.

- You can also use an aromatherapy diffuser with a scent that promotes thinking and concentration, such as citrus or peppermint.

Variations/adaptations/modifications: You can use a balloon instead of a ball.

Helpful hints/notes: Much of the setup for this activity can be done prior to gathering residents so that you are ready to begin once residents have gathered. Assemble all needed equipment and supplies prior to the start of the activity.

Evening Dementia Program

Target audience: Residents needing specialized dementia programming, and those with behavior issues, especially residents who typically exhibit "sundowning symptoms"

Objectives/outcomes:

- To provide tactile, auditory, olfactory, and visual stimulation and increase responsiveness

- To provide an opportunity for simple communication

- To promote relaxation, solace, pain management, and enjoyment

- To encourage interaction with others and increase social contact

- To decrease the frequency and severity of symptomatic behavior (tension, anxiety, and agitation)

- To stimulate the senses of withdrawn residents

- To soothe/relax residents who are agitated

- To improve relationships between caregivers and residents

- To help to induce sleep prior to bedtime

Recommended group size: Small, spending time one-on-one with each resident

Suggested time frame: 90 minutes (three 30-minute programs)

Special needs/ability level (physical/cognitive skills needed): Residents with varying levels of cognitive/physical abilities can join this group, as you work with them individually and provide needed assistance at their ability level. You need to make sure that residents are able to achieve some level of success in this activity for it to be beneficial to them.

Activity outline:

- After the evening meal, bring the residents into the multisensory room. If you do not have such a room, make the room as relaxing as possible with subdued lighting and minimal outside distractions. Place residents in a circle around the room.

- Have light or instrumental background music playing as they gather. This creates a calming, enveloping mood.

- Greet each resident by name and with a gentle touch or hug. Make sure residents are comfortable, which may mean placing them in more comfortable chairs than wheelchairs.

- For the first half-hour session, conduct a light physical activity (e.g., a recreational game such as basketball, ring toss, or beanbag toss), or have the residents move to music (with props). This helps them to wear off any remaining "energy" from the day.

- For the second half-hour session, change the music to relaxation music. During this time, set up the participants with multisensory room equipment. Then, offer a shoulder massage to each participant.

- Generally speaking, work on the shoulders and upper back; leave neck massages to the true therapists. Use hand sanitizer between each resident. Because you are not using lotion and are massaging the residents over their clothing, you do not have to wash your hands with soap and water between each resident, but you should do so periodically or if you come into contact with a resident's body fluids (e.g., drool). Next, move down the arms. Use a gentle kneading/squeezing action on the upper shoulders and rub gently downward on the resident's arms and down his or her spine if able. Rub the resident's back to the best of your ability while the resident is seated. Some residents may be able to lean forward slightly. If you are using a massager of some sort, apply only gentle pressure and move the massager in circular motions over the back and shoulders. Wilbarger protocol: helps reduce verbal and physical aggressive behavior. Using a soft brush, gently and slowly brush down the resident's arms, back, and legs. Repeat several times, while talking in a calm, soothing tone of voice. Then wrap the person in a weighted blanket (weighted blankets are commonly used in sensory rooms, as they provide a pleasant sensation of comfort when wrapped around the body).

- For the third and final half-hour session, lower the volume of the relaxation music and read short stories to the participants, interjecting simple questions to elicit responses and keep them focused. However, the goal of this program is to induce sleep

and a restful night. So, if residents drift off to sleep, that is great, as you have suc-
ceeded in achieving the goal.

- Use an aromatherapy diffuser with a scent that promotes relaxation, such as vanilla
or lavender, throughout the program.

Variations/adaptations/modifications: You have to adapt/modify your approach based
on the physical and cognitive ability level of each individual within the group. Go around and
provide the visual, verbal, and direct physical guidance that each person needs to be successful. Redirect as necessary. You will need to simplify tasks and offer more assistance to residents
with diminished abilities (they may be able to perform tasks with direct hand-over-hand guidance).

Helpful hints/notes: Observe all infection-control guidelines. Always keep in mind the
fragility of residents' skin and that they can bruise quite easily. Apply only the amount of
pressure that is comfortable and appropriate for them. Much of the setup for this activity can
be done prior to gathering residents so that you are ready to begin once residents have gathered. Assemble all needed equipment and supplies prior to the start of the activity. Clean and
disinfect activity supplies as needed/according to your facility's policy and procedure. Always
have a "Plan B" (and C, D, and E) for whatever programs you have planned for the evening
so that if residents do not respond positively to what is offered or if they lose interest, you are
ready to offer something else.

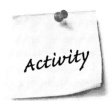

Activity | **Five Alive**

Target audience: Residents needing specialized dementia programming and those with behavior issues

Objectives/outcomes:

- To provide visual, tactile, auditory, and olfactory stimulation and increase responsiveness

- To provide an opportunity for simple communication

- To provide a pleasurable, failure-free and stress-free environment

- To allow individuals the time, space, and opportunity to enjoy the environment at their own pace, free from unrealistic expectations of others

- To promote relaxation, exploration, communication, and enjoyment

- To encourage interaction with others and increase social contact

- To decrease the frequency and severity of symptomatic behavior (tension, anxiety, and agitation)

- To stimulate the senses of withdrawn residents

- To soothe/relax residents who are agitated

- To enhance/increase attention span, thinking and reasoning skills, memory recall, and concentration

- To provide opportunities for emotional expression

- To improve mood by actively engaging residents at their level of ability

- To provide an atmosphere that encourages participants to explore their environment and to be able to enjoy themselves

- To promote the ability of participants to express themselves

- To promote person-centered care

- To improve relationships between caregivers and residents

Recommended group size: Small

Suggested time frame: 30 – 45 minutes

Special needs/ability level (physical/cognitive skills needed): Residents with varying levels of cognitive/physical abilities can join this group, as you set them up individually with objects at their ability level.

Activity outline:

- Have a portable sensory cart equipped with selected activity materials for varying degrees of cognitive loss (e.g., manipulatives, peg boards, lacing cards, nuts and bolts, PVC piping, music boxes, all-in-one activity boards, color dominoes, simple matching games, sound machines, light-up visuals, themed memory boxes/bags, things to touch, see, and smell, etc.).

- Residents will need to sit at tables for this activity.

- Play relaxing background music (auditory) and have aromatherapy, scented beads and a diffuser, scent stories, or a candle warmer with a candle (smell).

- Start out with a snack (taste).

- Set up each resident in attendance with an activity with which he or she can have some measure of success (tactile and visual). This requires that you have assessed the abilities and identified the needs, interests, and interventions of each resident in attendance.

- Work with each resident individually as needed, but let them do for themselves as much as they can and provide assistance only if it is truly needed.

- Rotate activities among the residents in attendance so that you can focus on stimulating different senses (hence the name "Five Alive"). You want to work on all senses to promote increased awareness of the environment, but only a few at a time so as not to be overstimulating and distracting.

Variations/adaptations/modifications: You have to adapt/modify your approach based on the physical and cognitive ability level of each individual within the group. Go around and provide the visual, verbal, and direct physical guidance that each person needs to be successful. Redirect as necessary. You will need to simplify tasks and offer more assistance to residents with diminished abilities (they may be able to perform tasks with direct hand-over-hand guidance).

Helpful hints/notes: Observe all infection-control guidelines and individual resident dietary needs/restrictions when serving food and beverages. Much of the setup for this activity can be done prior to gathering residents so that you are ready to begin once residents have gathered. Assemble all needed equipment and supplies prior to the start of the activity. Clean and disinfect activity supplies as needed/according to your facility's policy and procedure. State surveyors have loved this activity, as it provides individual attention and social contact, and it gets the residents actively engaged at their own level.

Folded Paper Paintings

Target audience: Residents needing specialized dementia programming and those with behavior issues

Objectives/outcomes:

- To provide visual and tactile stimulation and increase responsiveness.

- To provide an opportunity for simple communication.

- To promote communication and enjoyment.

- To encourage interaction with others and increase social contact.

- To enhance/increase attention span, thinking and reasoning skills, concentration, and identification of colors and shapes, and promote the ability to follow one-step direction.

- Allows residents to express their creative ideas. Promotes residents' self-esteem through successful projects. Maintains and develops fine motor skills and hand-eye coordination. Provides residents with an opportunity for choice and preference in regard to the finished project.

- To improve mood by actively engaging residents at their level of ability.

Recommended group size: Small; can also be done one-on-one in resident's room

Suggested time frame: 30 – 45 minutes

Special needs/ability level (physical/cognitive skills needed): Residents with varying levels of cognitive/physical abilities can join this group, as you work with them individually and provide needed assistance at their ability level. You need to make sure that residents are able to achieve some level of success in this activity for it to be beneficial to them.

Activity outline:

- You will need paper, scissors, old newspaper, and tempera paints.

- Have this be at least a monthly activity with a selected theme (e.g., holiday).

- Cover the work area with old newspaper to cut down on cleanup time.

- Discuss your theme with the group and explain what you will be doing. For example, "The next holiday is Easter. Today we are going to make colorful Easter eggs."

- Let residents choose their background color (offer a selection by showing them the colors that are available, but do not show them more than five choices). Once they have chosen the color of their paper, instruct them to cut the paper into any shape they choose.

- Next, have them choose the paint colors they want to use. Again, offer them visual choices, but limit the number of choices so as not to be too overwhelming. Provide them with one-step cues as you go along. If they are able, let them squirt small amounts of paint onto the paper; otherwise, the staff may squirt the paint onto the paper based on where the residents want the paint placed. If they are able, let them fold the paper in half and over again; otherwise, the staff may do that for them. Next, have them rub the folded-over paper for a period of time. Finally, tell them to open the paper and see their beautiful painting. Discuss with the group how everyone's painting is unique and ask what everyone likes about each one. Put the resident's name on the back of his or her painting, and hang it in a group display where the staff, family members, and other residents can enjoy it.

- Work with each resident individually as needed, but let them do for themselves as much as they can and provide assistance only if it is truly needed (you may need to point out a color and shape, but they may be able to cover it themselves).

- You can also use an aromatherapy diffuser with a scent that promotes mental stimulation, such as citrus or peppermint.

- You may play background music that promotes free expression (e.g., classical music).

Variations/adaptations/modifications: You have to adapt/modify your approach based on the cognitive ability level of each individual within the group. Go around and provide the visual, verbal, and direct physical guidance that each person needs to be successful. Redirect as necessary. You will need to offer more assistance to residents with diminished abilities. This requires that you have assessed the abilities and identified the needs, interests, and interventions of each resident in attendance. For a variation, you can have them add glitter while the paint is still wet. Another variation is to create a marble painting instead of folding over the paper. To do this, place each resident's piece of paper on a cookie sheet. Have the residents choose the paint colors they want to use. Again, offer them visual choices, but limit them so as not to be too overwhelming. Provide them with one-step cues as you go along. If they are able, let them squirt small amounts of paint onto the paper; otherwise, the staff may squirt the paint onto the paper based on where the residents want the paint placed. Place a half dozen marbles onto the cookie sheet. Tell the residents to roll the marbles around on their paper. (Rolling the marbles helps residents to work off aggression, and they find it mesmerizing; therefore, it is therapeutic in nature.) This will create interesting and varied designs. Discuss with the group how everyone's painting is unique and ask what everyone likes about each one. Put each resident's name on the back of his or her painting, and hang it in a group display where the staff, family members, and other residents can enjoy it.

Helpful hints/notes: Much of the setup for this activity can be done prior to gathering residents so that you are ready to begin once residents have gathered. Assemble all needed equipment and supplies prior to the start of the activity.

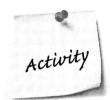

Activity

Grandma's Kitchen on a Cart

Target audience: Residents needing specialized dementia programming

Objectives/outcomes:

- To provide olfactory and gustatory stimulation and increase responsiveness

- To provide an opportunity for simple communication

- To provide a pleasurable, failure-free and stress-free environment

- To allow individuals the time, space, and opportunity to enjoy the environment at their own pace, free from unrealistic expectations of others

- To promote relaxation, exploration, communication, and enjoyment

- To encourage interaction with others and increase social contact

- To stimulate the senses of withdrawn residents

- To enhance/increase attention span, thinking and reasoning skills, memory recall, and concentration

- To provide opportunities for emotional expression

- To improve mood by actively engaging residents at their level of ability

- To provide an atmosphere that encourages participants to explore their environment and to be able to enjoy themselves

- To promote the ability of participants to express themselves

- To promote person-centered care

- To improve relationships between caregivers and residents

Recommended group size: Small

Suggested time frame: 30 – 45 minutes

Special needs/ability level (physical/cognitive skills needed): Residents with moderate cognitive impairments, and residents who can follow simple directions and complete simple, one-step tasks. You need to make sure that residents are able to achieve some level of success in this activity for it to be beneficial to them.

Activity outline:

- This is a very simple cooking/baking group for residents with dementia that is done in their familiar surroundings. It requires that you preselect a simple recipe for a treat that they can eat afterward, and that you have the needed supplies on hand (through the Dietary Department or by shopping for them).

- You will need a toaster/convection oven, cart, and bin with needed supplies.

- Do all prep work prior to starting the activity. Leave simple tasks for residents to perform.

- Recipes for "mixing in the bag" work great for this group as residents can more easily manipulate the mix in the bag than stir ingredients in a bowl.

- The recipe can be as simple as mixing pudding, mixing and baking packaged muffin, cake, or brownie mix, baking biscuits from a tube, or baking sweet rolls or cookies from a tube. The smell of the food baking is great aromatherapy. This in itself will encourage residents to see what is "cooking," and it stimulates the appetite in those who have a reduced appetite.

- Have a selected topic (the next holiday, the current season, etc.), and a simple discussion/reminiscence while the food is baking and while the group is tasting it afterward.

Variations/adaptations/modifications: You have to adapt/modify your approach based on the physical and cognitive ability level of each individual within the group. Go around and provide the visual, verbal, and direct physical guidance that each person needs to be successful. Redirect as necessary. You will need to simplify tasks and offer more assistance to residents with diminished abilities (they may be able to perform tasks with direct hand-over-hand guidance). You could read them a short story or look through recipe books while items are baking or being made, and while they are eating their treat instead of conducting a discussion group. Get them involved in the story by asking simple, direct questions regarding what you have read and get them to reminisce based on the story. You could also have a blender on the cart and create blended high-calorie nutritional beverages. A bread machine, waffle maker, and electric frying pan are additional options for cooking/baking on individual units outside the kitchen.

Helpful hints/notes: Observe all infection-control guidelines and individual resident dietary needs/restrictions when serving food and beverages. Much of the setup for this activity can be done prior to gathering residents so that you are ready to begin once residents have gathered. Assemble all needed equipment and supplies prior to the start of the activity. Toaster ovens, waffle makers, and electric frying pans are hot to the touch and can burn, so keep residents away from them for their own safety.

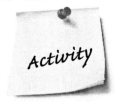

Hands Alive

Target audience: Residents needing specialized dementia programming and those with behavior issues

Objectives/outcomes:

- To provide tactile stimulation and increase responsiveness

- To provide an opportunity for simple communication

- To promote relaxation, solace, pain management, and enjoyment

- To encourage interaction with others and increase social contact

- To decrease the frequency and severity of symptomatic behavior (tension, anxiety, and agitation)

- To stimulate the senses of withdrawn residents

- To soothe/relax residents who are agitated

- To improve relationships between caregivers and residents

Recommended group size: One-on-one in residents' rooms, or in a small group going around one-on-one

Suggested time frame: Approximately five minutes per resident

Special needs/ability level (physical/cognitive skills needed): None

Activity outline:

- You will need a bucket/basin, clean washcloths and hand towels, nicely scented bath gel and hand lotion, hand sanitizing gel, a small disposable garbage bag for dirty linen (tie to cart handle), and a cart.

- This is not a hand washing activity. It is a hand massage technique using warm, wet, scented washcloths. Apply the hand sanitizing gel to your hands. Fill the basin with warm water and squirt a small amount of scented bath gel into the water. Gently massage each resident's hands with the washcloth (gently massage across the top of the hand and the palm, moving down and around each finger). The warm, moist cloth helps to relax the hand. Repeat with other hand. Next, gently pat the hands dry; apply a small amount of scented lotion to the hands and gently massage it in. During this time, talk about supportive RO (e.g., simple current events, the season, upcoming holidays, the weather, the resident's family, and things of interest to each individual resident). Also talk about what you are doing, and what you will be doing next. Ask the resident how the massage makes him or her feel and what the resident is thinking; this way, you are engaging the resident into the activity even if he or she is unable to respond verbally. Take note of any body language the resident may be exhibiting to indicate his or her pleasure or dislike.

- Dispose of the dirty linens in the garbage bag. Wash your hands. Move on to the next resident. You can expect to complete five to six massages in a 30-minute period.

- If you are doing this in a small group setting, play some relaxing background music.

- This is a great sensory activity to do in a multisensory room, but if you do not have such a room, make the room as relaxing as possible with subdued lighting and minimal outside distractions. Place residents in a circle around the room.

- Put the dirty linen bag in the dirty linen room. Disinfect the basin and cart when the activity is completed.

Helpful hints/notes: For infection control purposes, never place a used washcloth into the basin. You can use the basin of warm water for five to six residents, and then you will need to empty it and refill it with clean warm water.

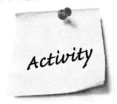

Hidden Treasures Sensory

Target audience: Residents needing specialized dementia programming and those with behavior issues

Objectives/outcomes:

- To provide visual and tactile stimulation and increase responsiveness

- To provide an opportunity for simple communication

- To promote communication and enjoyment

- To encourage interaction with others and increase social contact

- To enhance/increase attention span and memory recall, promote physical movement, and promote object identification, concentration, and reminiscence

- To promote relaxation

- To decrease the frequency and severity of symptomatic behavior (tension, anxiety, and agitation)

- To stimulate the senses of withdrawn residents

- To soothe/relax residents who are agitated

- To improve relationships between caregivers and residents

- To improve mood by actively engaging residents at their level of ability

Recommended group size: Small or one-on-one

Suggested time frame: 30 minutes

Special needs/ability level (physical/cognitive skills needed): Residents with varying levels of cognitive/physical abilities can join this group, as you work with them individually and provide needed assistance at their ability level. They need to be able to identify objects by touching them. You need to make sure that residents are able to achieve some level of success in this activity for it to be beneficial to them.

Activity outline:

- You will need a variety of objects that are easily identified through touch, as well as a pillowcase or tote bag in which to "hide" the objects.

- Place one object inside the pillowcase and have residents reach in and feel the object without looking. Give each resident a chance to feel the object and then ask each resident whether he or she can tell you what the object is. Show the resident the object and discuss its use before moving on to the next object.

- It's best to use everyday small objects (e.g., pen or pencil, eraser, book, spool of thread, clothespin, brush/comb, ball, plastic cup, wooden spoon, ruler, toothbrush, alarm clock, tea bag, tea ball, apple, banana, deck of cards, etc.).

- You can also use an aromatherapy diffuser with a scent that promotes thinking and concentration, such as citrus or peppermint.

Variations/adaptations/modifications: A variation of this activity is to put three familiar everyday objects on a tray, have residents identify them, and talk about each item for a few minutes (e.g., its use). Then remove one item and ask them whether they can tell you what item you removed from the tray. If they need something more challenging, remove all the items and ask them to identify them; as they get them right, place them back on the tray.

Helpful hints/notes: Much of the setup for this activity can be done prior to gathering residents so that you are ready to begin once residents have gathered. Assemble all needed equipment and supplies prior to the start of the activity.

Match Game

Target audience: Residents needing specialized dementia programming

Objectives/outcomes:

- To provide visual and tactile stimulation and increase responsiveness

- To provide an opportunity for simple communication

- To promote communication and enjoyment

- To encourage interaction with others and increase social contact

- To enhance/increase attention span and memory recall, thinking and reasoning skills, concentration, and identification of numbers and card suits, and promote the ability to follow one-step directions

- To improve mood by actively engaging residents at their level of ability

Recommended group size: Small if the residents need extensive assistance, large if some residents within the group are able to participate unassisted

Suggested time frame: 30 – 45 minutes

Special needs/ability level (physical/cognitive skills needed): Residents with the cognitive capacity to identify card suits and/or numbers and follow one-step directions. Residents with varying levels of cognitive/physical abilities can join this group, as you work with them individually and provide needed assistance at their ability level. You need to make sure that residents are able to achieve some level of success in this activity for it to be beneficial to them.

Activity outline:

- You will need many decks of standard-size playing cards (mixed together), plus an extra-large deck for the caller. This is a card bingo game.

- Pass out five cards face up in front of each resident. (It does not matter what they are or whether each resident has more than one card of the same number and/or suit.)

Explain that you will be calling out the card and suit from your deck of cards, and that if they have that card they are to turn it over. The first person to have all five cards turned over is to call out "Match!" and wins the game. You may award prizes, but it is not necessary. Your goal is to have residents identify numbers and suits.

- Work with each resident individually as needed, but let them do for themselves as much as they can and provide assistance only if it is truly needed (you may need to point out a card, but they may be able to turn it over themselves).

- You can also use an aromatherapy diffuser with a scent that promotes mental stimulation, such as citrus or peppermint.

- Provide the visual cue—showing the large card—and the verbal cue—stating the card number and suit. Repeat as needed to allow them to flip their card over if they have it.

Variations/adaptations/modifications: You have to adapt/modify your approach based on the cognitive ability level of each individual within the group. Go around and provide the visual, verbal, and direct physical guidance that each person needs to be successful. Redirect as necessary. You will need to offer more assistance to residents with diminished abilities (they may be able to perform tasks with direct hand-over-hand guidance). This requires that you have assessed the abilities and identified the needs, interests, and interventions of each resident in attendance.

Helpful hints/notes: Many casinos will give you free decks of cards for the asking. Much of the setup for this activity can be done prior to gathering residents so that you are ready to begin once residents have gathered. Assemble all needed equipment and supplies prior to the start of the activity.

Memory Matching

Target audience: Residents needing specialized dementia programming and those with behavior issues

Objectives/outcomes:

- To provide visual and tactile stimulation and increase responsiveness

- To provide an opportunity for simple communication

- To promote communication and enjoyment

- To encourage interaction with others and increase social contact

- To enhance/increase attention span and memory recall, thinking, reasoning and concentration skills, object identification, and matching skills

- To decrease the frequency and severity of symptomatic behavior (tension, anxiety, and agitation)

- To stimulate the senses of withdrawn residents

- To improve mood by actively engaging residents at their level of ability

Recommended group size: One-on-one

Suggested time frame: 15 – 20 minutes

Special needs/ability level (physical/cognitive skills needed): Residents with varying levels of cognitive/physical abilities can join this group, as you work with them individually and provide needed assistance at their ability level. They need to be able to identify objects and find matching pairs. You need to make sure that residents are able to achieve some level of success in this activity for it to be beneficial to them.

Activity outline:

- You will need pairs of pictures of everyday objects that you have taken and printed ahead of time. (Pictures of everyday objects are generally more successful because they most likely will be familiar to residents.) Some suggested everyday objects include toothbrushes, bars of soap, books, pencils, pads of paper, TVs, radios, clocks, chairs, tables, stoves, refrigerators, sofas, beds, pillows, folded blankets, towels, laundry soap, brooms, vacuums, dust pans, rugs, plants, pictures, dolls, dogs, cats, babies, girls, boys, men, women, and mailboxes.

• Lay out the pairs of pictures for the resident to see, and have him or her identify and talk about each picture to help get the image set in his or her mind. Next, turn the pictures over, mix them up, and have the resident turn over two pictures at a time. The resident is looking to find a matching pair. When the resident finds a matching pair, those cards remain face up. The number of pairs that you have the resident try to match varies with each individual's ability level. Try with two pairs and work your way up so that the resident achieves success in the beginning and the task becomes more challenging as he or she progresses. When the resident starts to demonstrate decreased ability, you will know that you have exceeded the resident's abilities and that you need to take the activity back to a level that is challenging, yet allows for some success.

• Work with each resident individually as needed, but let them do for themselves as much as they can and provide assistance only if it is truly needed (you may need to prompt their memory, but they may be able to turn the cards over themselves).

• You can also use an aromatherapy diffuser with a scent that promotes thinking and concentration, such as citrus or peppermint.

Variations/adaptations/modifications: You have to adapt/modify your approach based on the cognitive ability level of each individual. Provide the visual, verbal, and direct physical guidance that each person needs to be successful. Redirect as necessary. You will need to offer more assistance to residents with diminished abilities. This requires that you have assessed the abilities and identified the needs, interests, and interventions of each resident in attendance.

Helpful hints/notes: Much of the setup for this activity can be done prior to gathering residents so that you are ready to begin once residents have gathered. Assemble all needed equipment and supplies prior to the start of the activity.

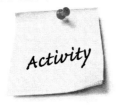

Morning Wakeup Sensory Program

Target audience: Residents needing specialized dementia programming and those with behavior issues

Objectives/outcomes:

- To provide tactile, auditory, visual, and olfactory stimulation and increase responsiveness

- To provide an opportunity for simple communication

- To promote relaxation, solace, pain management, and enjoyment

- To encourage interaction with others and increase social contact

- To decrease the frequency and severity of symptomatic behavior (tension, anxiety, and agitation)

- To stimulate the senses of withdrawn residents

- To soothe/relax residents who are agitated

- To improve relationships between caregivers and residents

Recommended group size: One-on-one in resident rooms, or a small group working with each resident one-on-one

Suggested time frame: Approximately five minutes per resident

Special needs/ability level (physical/cognitive skills needed): Residents with varying levels of cognitive/physical abilities can join this group, as you work with them individually and provide needed assistance at their ability level. You need to make sure that residents are able to achieve some level of success in this activity for it to be beneficial to them.

Activity outline:

- After breakfast, bring the residents into the multisensory room. If you do not have such a room, make the room as relaxing as possible with subdued lighting and

- minimal outside distractions. Place residents in a circle around the room.

- Have soft, relaxing background music playing as they gather. This creates a calming, enveloping mood.

- Greet each resident by name and with a gentle touch or hug. You can also "swaddle" them in blankets (or weighted blankets) as this helps them feel secure. Make sure residents are comfortable, which may mean placing them in more comfortable chairs than wheelchairs.

- Start by softly shaping the day with a series of activities. Gently brush their hair, apply lotion to their hands, face, and feet using a gentle massaging touch, and play nature videos with soothing background music. Utilize some of the multisensory room materials, or a multisensory cart of supplies, working individually with each participant.

- Provide residents with supportive RO while working with them (talk about the weather, the present season, upcoming holidays, current happenings in the nursing home, their family, etc.).

- You can also use an aromatherapy diffuser with a scent that promotes relaxation, such as vanilla or lavender, or a seasonal scent (spices or cinnamon for winter; rain, or lily of the valley, lilacs, or hyacinths for spring; watermelon or roses for summer; and pumpkin or apples and cinnamon for fall).

Variations/adaptations/modifications: You have to adapt/modify your approach based on the physical and cognitive ability level of each individual within the group. Go around and provide the visual, verbal, and direct physical guidance that each person needs to be successful. Redirect as necessary. You will need to simplify tasks and offer more assistance to residents with diminished abilities (they may be able to perform tasks with direct hand-over-hand guidance).

Helpful hints/notes: Observe all infection-control guidelines. Much of the setup for this activity can be done prior to gathering residents so that you are ready to begin once residents have gathered. Assemble all needed equipment and supplies prior to the start of each activity. Clean and disinfect the activity supplies as needed according to your facility's policy and procedure.

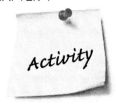

Music with Movement Program for the Memory/Sensory Program

Target audience: Residents with cognitive impairments (moderate to severe). This is meant to be a morning activity to engage the residents in their day.

Objectives/outcomes:

- To provide visual, auditory, and tactile stimulation and increase responsiveness

- To provide an opportunity for simple communication

- To provide a pleasurable, failure-free and stress-free environment

- To allow individuals the time, space, and opportunity to enjoy the environment at their own pace, free from unrealistic expectations of others

- To promote large motor physical activity, communication, and enjoyment

- To encourage interaction with others and increase social contact

- To enhance/increase attention span and concentration and promote the ability to follow one-step directions or mimic desired actions

- To improve mood by actively engaging residents at their level of ability

- To provide an atmosphere that encourages participants to explore their environment and to be able to enjoy themselves

- To promote the ability of participants to express themselves

- To promote person-centered care

- To improve relationships between caregivers and residents

Recommended group size: Small (8 – 12)

Suggested time frame: Approximately 30 minutes

Special needs/ability level (physical/cognitive skills needed): Residents with the physical capacity to follow one-step directions or mimic desired actions. You need to make sure that residents are able to achieve some level of success in this activity for it to be beneficial to them.

Activity outline:

- Gather needed supplies before gathering the residents. You will need music (some songs with a slow tempo and some with an upbeat tempo), a CD player, rhythm instruments, and exercise props (e.g., scarves, noodles, pinwheels, etc.).

- Seat residents in a circle or semicircle. Start out by welcoming everyone to the group, and greeting them by name, shaking their hand, and saying "Good morning." Tell them you will be listening to music for enjoyment and will move to the music (free-form style).

- Begin with music that is mellow and has a slow rhythm, preferably a familiar song that residents can sing to if desired. Hand out the rhythm instruments. The group leader should keep the beat with a drum or rhythm sticks. Simple verbal and visual cues should be given. Use mirroring techniques and hand-over-hand/direct physical guidance for those who require this, moving around from resident to resident to give the one-on-one attention that is needed. Provide praise throughout. Always observe the residents for their responses to this activity. (Often, when you move on to someone else, a resident will continue to perform a repetitive task.) Move to two or three mellow songs in the beginning (Carly Simon's "Into White" is a great CD for this part of the activity).

- Stop the music and replace it with music that has an upbeat tempo. Continue using the rhythm instruments (either the same ones, or residents can exchange instruments with each other). Jazz, blues, or Dixieland music is ideal for this part of the activity, which should pick up the pace and comprise three or four songs.

- Switch back to mellower music and hand out the exercise props. Encourage freeform movement, use the mirroring technique, and promote ROM. Do this for two or three songs.

- Switch to mellow songs for the close of the activity. Collect all the props. Seat the residents so that they can join hands, and have the leader join hands as well. Make eye contact with each resident. Promote the singing of songs. Sway to the music, and bring the residents down to a relaxed mood once again. Do this for one or two songs.

This is intended to promote inclusion, human touch, and social connections.

- Thank everyone for joining in and participating in the group.

Variations/adaptations/modifications: You have to adapt/modify your approach based on the physical and cognitive ability level of each individual within the group. Go around and provide the visual, verbal, and direct physical guidance that each person needs to be successful. Redirect as necessary. You will need to offer more assistance to residents with diminished abilities (they may be able to perform tasks with direct hand-over-hand guidance). This requires that you have assessed the abilities and identified the needs, interests, and interventions of each resident in attendance.

Helpful hints/notes: Much of the setup for this activity can be done prior to gathering residents so that you are ready to begin once residents have gathered. Assemble all needed equipment and supplies prior to the start of the activity.

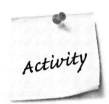

Activity **Name Five**

Target audience: Residents needing specialized dementia programming and those with behavior issues

Objectives/outcomes:

- To provide an opportunity for simple communication

- To promote communication and enjoyment

- To encourage interaction with others and increase social contact

- To enhance/increase attention span and memory recall, thinking, reasoning and concentration skills, and reminiscence

- To decrease the frequency and severity of symptomatic behavior (tension, anxiety, and agitation)

- To stimulate the senses of withdrawn residents

- To improve mood by actively engaging residents at their level of ability

Recommended group size: Small or one-on-one

Suggested time frame: 30 minutes

Special needs/ability level (physical/cognitive skills needed): Residents with varying levels of cognitive/physical abilities can join this group, as you work with them individually and provide needed assistance at their ability level. They need to be able to identify items within categories. You need to make sure that residents are able to achieve some level of success in this activity for it to be beneficial to them.

Activity outline:

- The object of Name Five is for residents to work as a group (or individually) to come up with five objects within each category.

- Start your statement like this: "Name five [name of category]."

THE BIG BOOK OF RESIDENT ACTIVITIES

181

4

ACTIVITIES FOR RESIDENTS WITH DEMENTIA, ALZHEIMER'S, AND BEHAVIORAL ISSUES

- Sample categories for this game include fruits, vegetables, makes of cars, animals, plants, flowers, trees, girls' names, boys' names, sports, hobbies, toys, meats, desserts, candies, soups, pies, cookies, cakes, ice cream flavors, letters of the alphabet, occupations, cities, states, countries, presidents, school subjects, kids' games, items you would see in a beauty shop, things found in a kitchen (or bathroom, bedroom, living room, garage, at the beach, in a hardware store, in a grocery store, at a restaurant, or in a doctor's office), places you could go for vacation, articles of clothing, ways to make potatoes, household tasks, things a secretary might do, modes of transportation, famous people, famous places, holidays, colors, shapes, and types of weather.

- Work with each resident individually as needed, but let them do for themselves as much as they can and provide assistance only if it is truly needed (you may ask them a question to help them think of an answer or provide additional clues).

- You can also use an aromatherapy diffuser with a scent that promotes thinking and concentration, such as citrus or peppermint.

Variations/adaptations/modifications: You have to adapt/modify your approach based on the cognitive ability level of each individual. Provide the visual, verbal, and direct physical guidance that each person needs to be successful. Redirect as necessary. You will need to offer more assistance to residents with diminished abilities. This requires that you have assessed the abilities and identified the needs, interests, and interventions of each resident in attendance.

Helpful hints/notes: Much of the setup for this activity can be done prior to gathering residents so that you are ready to begin once residents have gathered. Assemble all needed equipment and supplies prior to the start of the activity.

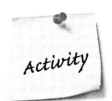
Activity

Noodle Ball

Target audience: Residents needing specialized dementia programming

Objectives/outcomes:

- To provide visual and tactile stimulation and increase responsiveness

- To provide an opportunity for simple communication

- To provide a pleasurable, failure-free and stress-free environment

- To allow individuals the time, space, and opportunity to enjoy the environment at their own pace, free from unrealistic expectations of others

- To promote large motor physical activity and upper-body range of motion, communication, and enjoyment

- To encourage interaction with others and increase social contact

- To enhance/increase attention span, thinking and reasoning skills, and concentration, and promote the ability to follow one-step directions or mimic desired actions

- To improve mood by actively engaging residents at their level of ability

- To provide an atmosphere that encourages participants to explore their environment and to be able to enjoy themselves

- To promote the ability of participants to express themselves

- To promote person-centered care

- To improve relationships between caregivers and residents

Recommended group size: Small

Suggested time frame: 30 minutes

Special needs/ability level (physical/cognitive skills needed): Residents with the physical capacity to hold the noodle in one hand, to hit/bat at the balloon, and to follow one-step directions or mimic desired actions. You need to make sure that residents are able to achieve some level of success in this activity for it to be beneficial to them.

Activity outline:

- You will need enough swim noodles for each participating resident. Cut each noodle in half. You also need an inflated balloon (the bigger the better, but must be light in weight).

- Form two teams by placing residents in rows as you would for volleyball (without a net). Allow adequate spacing between participants. Give each resident a noodle. Explain to them that they are to bat at the balloon and try to keep it up in the air for as long as they can. You will toss the balloon up in the air for them. You can keep score if you desire, but that is not necessary. Simply encouraging them to see how long they can keep the balloon in the air is challenging and rewarding enough in most cases.

- Work with each resident individually as needed, but let them do for themselves as much as they can and provide assistance only if it is truly needed.

- Play some background music that will promote physical activity (rag time, marching band, etc.).

- You can also use an aromatherapy diffuser with a scent that promotes physical activity and mental stimulation, such as citrus or peppermint.

Variations/adaptations/modifications: You have to adapt/modify your approach based on the physical and cognitive ability level of each individual within the group. Go around and provide the visual, verbal, and direct physical guidance that each person needs to be successful. Redirect as necessary. You will need to offer more assistance to residents with diminished abilities (they may be able to perform tasks with direct hand-over-hand guidance). This requires that you have assessed the abilities and identified the needs, interests, and interventions of each resident in attendance.

Helpful hints/notes: Buy swim noodles at the end of the summer season to save money. Much of the setup for this activity can be done prior to gathering residents so that you are ready to begin once residents have gathered. Assemble all needed equipment and supplies prior to the start of the activity. Clean and disinfect the activity supplies as needed according to your facility's policy and procedure.

Noodle Exercise

Target audience: Residents needing specialized dementia programming

Objectives/outcomes:

- To provide visual and tactile stimulation and increase responsiveness

- To provide an opportunity for simple communication

- To provide a pleasurable, failure-free and stress-free environment

- To allow individuals the time, space, and opportunity to enjoy the environment at their own pace, free from unrealistic expectations of others

- To promote large motor physical activity and upper-body range of motion, communication, and enjoyment

- To encourage interaction with others and increase social contact

- To enhance/increase attention span, thinking and reasoning skills, and concentration, and promote the ability to follow one-step directions or mimic desired actions

- To improve mood by actively engaging residents at their level of ability

- To provide an atmosphere that encourages participants to explore their environment and to be able to enjoy themselves

- To promote the ability of participants to express themselves

- To promote person-centered care

- To improve relationships between caregivers and residents

Recommended group size: Small

Suggested time frame: 30 minutes

Special needs/ability level (physical/cognitive skills needed): Residents with the physical capacity to hold a noodle in one hand and to follow one-step directions or mimic desired actions. You need to make sure that residents are able to achieve some level of success in this activity for it to be beneficial to them.

Activity outline:

- You will need enough swim noodles for each participating resident and staff member. Cut each noodle in half.

- Work with each resident individually as needed, but let them do for themselves as much as they can and provide assistance only if it is truly needed.

- Play some background music that will promote physical activity (ragtime, marching band, etc.).

- You can also use an aromatherapy diffuser with a scent that promotes physical activity and mental stimulation, such as citrus or peppermint.

- Demonstrate desired actions (visual cues) and provide one-step verbal instructions for each desired action.

- Start by having the residents hold a swim noodle in both hands horizontally to the floor at chest level (if they are able) and out in front of them. If a resident has had a stroke and cannot hold the noodle in this manner, have the resident use his or her unaffected side. Have the residents raise their noodles as high over their heads as they can, lower them to their waists, and then lower them some more, going as low as they can. Repeat each sequence five to 10 times as repetitive activities are great for residents with dementia, and they may require several tries before they get the hang of it. Always perform each movement slowly and deliberately. Next, have them form their noodle into a circle and move it as though it is a steering wheel. Next, have them hold it out in front of them at chest level and ask them to march in place, bringing their knees up to the noodle if they are able. Next, have them swing the noodle from side to side (like a tap dancer would; you may think of and add other movements with the noodle being held in both hands). Once you have completed the movements holding the noodle in both hands, switch to having them hold the noodle with one hand. (Do not use the words *left* and *right* in your directions; simply tell them to "switch to the other hand". If they can use only one hand, tell them to continue with that hand. It also helps to use verbal cues that further define what you want them to do; for example, "Let's conduct an orchestra," etc.). Some one-handed movements include tapping your toes with the noodle to the beat of the music, pretending you are conducting an orchestra, creating figure eights, raising your arms up high and then down to the ground, making small and then large circles (both in front and to the sides), and swinging the noodle from side to side. (Again, you may think of and add other movements while holding the noodle in one hand.)

Variations/adaptations/modifications: You have to adapt/modify your approach based on the physical and cognitive ability level of each individual within the group. Go around and provide the visual, verbal, and direct physical guidance that each person needs to be successful. Redirect as necessary. You will need to offer more assistance to residents with diminished abilities (they may be able to perform tasks with direct hand-over-hand guidance). This requires that you have assessed the abilities and identified the needs, interests, and interventions of each resident in attendance.

Helpful hints/notes: Buy swim noodles at the end of the summer season to save money. Much of the setup for this activity can be done prior to gathering residents so that you are ready to begin once residents have gathered. Assemble all needed equipment and supplies prior to the start of the activity. Clean and disinfect the activity supplies as needed according to your facility's policy and procedure.

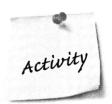

Activity

Object Identification

Target audience: Residents needing specialized dementia programming and those with behavior issues

Objectives/outcomes:

- To provide an opportunity for simple communication

- To promote communication and enjoyment

- To encourage interaction with others and increase social contact

- To enhance/increase attention span, thinking, reasoning and concentration skills, object identification, and reminiscence

- To decrease the frequency and severity of symptomatic behavior (tension, anxiety, and agitation)

- To stimulate the senses of withdrawn residents

- To improve mood by actively engaging residents at their level of ability

Recommended group size: Small or one-on-one

Suggested time frame: 30 minutes

Special needs/ability level (physical/cognitive skills needed): Residents with varying levels of cognitive/physical abilities can join this group, as you work with them individually and provide needed assistance at their ability level. They need to be able to identify objects. You need to make sure that residents are able to achieve some level of success in this activity for it to be beneficial to them.

Activity outline:

- You will need to take pictures of ordinary, everyday objects or purchase ready-made cards.

- Here is a list of ordinary, everyday objects to get you started: fruits, vegetables, cars, animals, plants, flowers, trees, sports equipment, hobby supplies, toys, toothbrushes, bars of soap, books, pencils, pads of paper, TVs, radios, clocks, chairs, tables, stoves, refrigerators, sofas, beds, pillows, folded blankets, towels, laundry soap, brooms, vacuums, dust pans, rugs, plants, pictures, dolls, dogs, cats, babies, girls, boys, men, women, mailboxes, toilets (humor is good), silverware, dishes, pots and pans, and lawn mowers. (Just walk around your house, garage, and yard and snap pictures.)

- The object is to have the residents look at the pictures and identify what they see. Ask open-ended questions to promote discussion (e.g., if they identify the toilet, ask them whether they remember a time when toilets were not everyday household items; this should prompt some interesting discussions about outhouses).

- Work with each resident individually as needed, but let them do for themselves as much as they can and provide assistance only if it is truly needed (you may ask them a question to help them think of an answer or provide additional clues).

- You can also use an aromatherapy diffuser with a scent that promotes thinking and concentration, such as citrus or peppermint.

Variations/adaptations/modifications: You have to adapt/modify your approach based on the cognitive ability level of each individual. Provide the visual, verbal, and direct physical guidance that each person needs to be successful. Redirect as necessary. You will need to offer more assistance to residents with diminished abilities. This requires that you have assessed the abilities and identified the needs, interests, and interventions of each resident in attendance.

Helpful hints/notes: Much of the setup for this activity can be done prior to gathering residents so that you are ready to begin once residents have gathered. Assemble all needed equipment and supplies prior to the start of the activity.

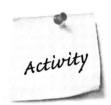

Activity **Parachute Fun**

Target audience: Residents needing specialized dementia programming and those with behavior issues

Objectives/outcomes:

- To provide visual stimulation and increase responsiveness

- To provide an opportunity for simple communication

- To promote communication and enjoyment

- To encourage interaction with others and increase social contact

- To enhance/increase attention span, and promote physical movement/large motor skills and range of motion

- To decrease the frequency and severity of symptomatic behavior (tension, anxiety, and agitation)

- To stimulate the senses of withdrawn residents

- To improve mood by actively engaging residents at their level of ability

Recommended group size: Small (enough to fit around the parachute, so it depends on the size of the parachute)

Suggested time frame: 30 minutes

Special needs/ability level (physical/cognitive skills needed): Residents with varying levels of cognitive/physical abilities can join the group, as you work with them individually and provide needed assistance at their ability level. You need to make sure that residents are able to achieve some level of success in this activity for it to be beneficial to them.

Activity outline:

- You will need a parachute, ball, and other lightweight objects (e.g., plastic chickens, plastic fish, or balloons) to place on the parachute to make it more interesting.

- Set residents up in a circle around the parachute. Have them grasp the parachute in both hands (if they are able; otherwise, have them use their good hand).

- Place an object(s) on the parachute.

- Play lively music in the background.

- Have them move the parachute up and down to bounce the object(s) and see how high they can get the object(s) to bounce, yet remain on the parachute.

- Have the residents move the parachute in other ways as well (e.g., one side up and one side down, and back and forth). Have them do the "wave." Have them lift the parachute high and then low, roll a ball around the outer edges, and so on.

- Change the objects from time to time to keep it interesting.

Variations/adaptations/modifications: You can use a bed sheet if you do not have a parachute. The advantages of a parachute are the handles for them to hold on to and the colorfulness.

Helpful hints/notes: Much of the setup for this activity can be done prior to gathering residents so that you are ready to begin once residents have gathered. Assemble all needed equipment and supplies prior to the start of the activity.

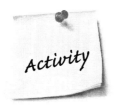

Activity   **Pet Therapy/Pet Visits**

Target audience: Residents who have an expressed interest in animals based on assessed interests. Dementia residents in particular respond positively to this program.

Objectives/outcomes:

- To offer residents the opportunity to enjoy contact and closeness with animals

- To provide the visual, tactile, and emotional stimulation that animals evoke

- To provide educational programs and environmental awareness

- To provide the TLC that pets afford

- To provide an opportunity for simple communication

- To promote communication and enjoyment

- To encourage interaction with others and increase social contact

- To improve mood by actively engaging residents at their level of ability

Recommended group size: One-on-one; small

Suggested time frame: 30 minutes per group (visits last about 10 – 15 minutes)

Special needs/ability level (physical/cognitive skills needed): Residents with all levels and abilities can join in this activity.

Activity outline:

- Place a towel onto the resident's lap or bed so that the animal does not touch the resident's clothing/bed

- Try to bring animals around to each resident to see, touch, hold, pet, brush, feed, and so on

- Discuss pets they may have had while they are holding/petting the animal

- Close the activity with a "Goodbye" and "Thank you"

- Complete hand washing with residents using hand wipes and/or an alcohol-based foam

Variations/adaptations/modifications: Pets can include dogs, cats, bunnies, and other animals such as hamsters. You can also include a registered therapy dog, facility pet, Humane Society animal, resident pets, and staff members' pets.

Helpful hints/notes: Check for allergies to animals before exposing a resident to the pet in the program. Also check with residents about their desire to be included in this program, as not everyone is comfortable with pets and some people have fears of certain animals. Much of the setup for this activity can be done prior to gathering residents so that you are ready to begin once residents have gathered. Assemble all needed equipment and supplies prior to the start of the activity.

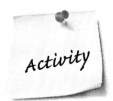

Activity

Picture Postcard Memories

Target audience: Residents needing specialized dementia programming

Objectives/outcomes:

- To provide visual stimulation and increase responsiveness

- To provide an opportunity for simple communication and reminiscence

- To promote communication and enjoyment

- To encourage interaction with others and increase social contact

- To enhance/increase attention span and memory recall, thinking and reasoning skills, concentration, and identification of objects, and promote the ability to follow one-step direction

- To improve mood by actively engaging residents at their level of ability

Recommended group size: Small or one-on-one

Suggested time frame: 30 minutes

Special needs/ability level (physical/cognitive skills needed): Residents with the cognitive capacity to identify pictures and answer simple questions. Residents with varying levels of cognitive/physical abilities can join this group, as you work with them individually and provide needed assistance at their ability level. You need to make sure that residents are able to achieve some level of success in this activity for it to be beneficial to them.

Activity outline:

- You will need picture postcards.

- Show one postcard at a time. Let each resident look at it for a period of time. Ask simple, direct questions to prompt discussion of each postcard—for example, "What do you see in the picture? Have you ever traveled here? Did you travel when you were younger? What did you like about traveling? Who did you travel with?" Ask other questions regarding what is in each picture and in response to residents' answers.

- You can also use an aromatherapy diffuser with a scent that promotes mental stimulation, such as citrus or peppermint.

Variations/adaptations/modifications: You have to adapt/modify your approach based on the cognitive ability level of each individual within the group. Go around and provide the visual, verbal, and direct physical guidance that each person needs to be successful. Redirect as necessary. You will need to offer more assistance to residents with diminished abilities. This requires that you have assessed the abilities and identified the needs, interests, and interventions of each resident in attendance. A variation of this activity is to use resident-specific postcards from their own travels. Another variation is to have duplicates of the cards and have residents match them up, providing them with enough choices to be stimulating and challenging, but not so overwhelming that it would be impossible for them to have some measure of success (e.g., two or three pairs of matches for someone with advanced dementia; or show a resident three pictures, two of which match, and ask the resident which picture doesn't belong). You can ask residents with moderate dementia to try to match five or six pairs.

Helpful hints/notes: You can buy postcards in your travels, or use postcards highlighting your area or region, as that is what residents will be most familiar with. You also can purchase postcards from activity supply catalogs. Much of the setup for this activity can be done prior to gathering residents so that you are ready to begin once residents have gathered. Assemble all needed equipment and supplies prior to the start of the activity.

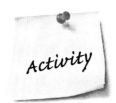

Activity

Recreational Programs

(Includes table games, puzzles, board games, basketball, ring toss, horseshoes, beanbag games and others)

Target audience: Residents who enjoy these types of programs based on assessed interests and needs; can include low-functioning residents

Objectives/outcomes:

- To provide recreational programs/opportunities for residents

- To provide long-term memory evoking programs

- To promote fine and gross motor skills and hand-eye coordination

- To offer competitive experiences

- To develop friendships among peers with similar activity interests

- To provide opportunities for fun, smiles, and laughter

- To promote reminiscence, mental stimulation, long-term memory skills, and cognitive/thinking skills

- To provide a learning opportunity

- To provide opportunities for physical exercise and friendly competition in a recreational setting

- To develop a sense of pride and self-esteem associated with friendly competition and team play

Recommended group size: *One-on-one, or small, medium, or large group

Suggested time frame: 30 – 60 minutes

Special needs/ability level (physical/cognitive skills needed): Medium to high functioning levels; low-functioning residents can participate with additional guidance and adaptations from the staff. Ability to follow directions, complete tasks, respond verbally, and interact on some level.

Activity outline:

- Organize and set out materials. Ensure that there are enough materials for all residents.

- Seat residents around tables or in a circle, depending on the activity.

- Introduce residents to each other.

- Make sure the room lighting and temperature are adequate and comfortable.

- Play soft instrumental music, if appropriate.

- Explain the recreational program's procedures or rules.

- Praise and thank residents for their participation.

- Award prizes or announce winners, as desired.

Variations/adaptations/modifications: *Some of the activities may be offered one-on-one for residents who are unwilling or unable to participate in a group. You will need to simplify tasks, make adaptations (residents may need closer targets, or verbal and visual cues), and offer more assistance to residents with diminished abilities (they may be able to perform tasks with direct hand-over-hand guidance). Some activities can include low-functioning residents when adaptations/modifications are made. Explain the recreational program's procedures or rules. Offer assistance as needed. Couple high-functioning residents with low-functioning residents. Repeat the rules as needed. Offer large-print materials to the visually impaired. Place hard-of-hearing residents near the speaker.

Helpful hints/notes: *When conducting this activity one-on-one, the activities staff and/or a trained volunteer can offer the activity to in-room residents who have an interest in such a program. A hand-held basket or rolling cart is a convenient way to transport materials to residents' rooms. When giving out prizes (for games), observe all dietary restrictions. Much of the setup for this activity can be done prior to gathering residents so that you are ready to begin once residents have gathered. Assemble all needed equipment and supplies prior to the start of the activity.

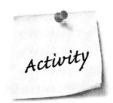

Activity

Relaxation Music with Movement for Sensory Program

Target audience: Residents with cognitive impairments who exhibit anxious or agitated behavior symptoms or sundowning. It is best to conduct this activity prior to those behaviors being exhibited. It is a great program for late afternoon (3 p.m. to 4 p.m.), or after supper. This activity is known to prevent or reduce behavioral symptoms.

Objectives/outcomes:

- To provide visual, auditory, and tactile stimulation and increase responsiveness

- To provide an opportunity for simple communication

- To provide a pleasurable, failure-free and stress-free environment

- To allow individuals the time, space, and opportunity to enjoy the environment at their own pace, free from unrealistic expectations of others

- To promote large motor physical activity, communication, and enjoyment

- To encourage interaction with others and increase social contact

- To enhance/increase attention span and concentration, and promote the ability to follow one-step directions or mimic desired actions

- To improve mood by actively engaging residents at their level of ability

- To provide an atmosphere that encourages participants to explore their environment and to be able to enjoy themselves

- To promote the ability of participants to express themselves

- To promote person-centered care

- To improve relationships between caregivers and residents

Recommended group size: Small (6 – 8)

Suggested time frame: 30 to 40 minutes

Special needs/ability level (physical/cognitive skills needed): Residents with the physical capacity to follow one-step directions or mimic desired actions. You need to make sure that residents are able to achieve some level of success in this activity for it to be beneficial to them.

Activity outline:

- Gather needed supplies before gathering the residents. You will need a CD player, calming music that is familiar to the target population, but that has a moderate rhythm and tempo, aromatherapy oils (lavender and vanilla are known to be relaxing scents), and a diffuser. Start the diffuser and music prior to gathering the residents to create a calming atmosphere.

- Greet each participant by name once the group is gathered. A circle or semicircle formation is good for this activity.

- Start with gentle, warm-up body movements. Use simple, direct statements when explaining what you want the residents to do, and provide visual cues as needed. Some participants may need one-on-one attention with direct physical guidance. Focus on large motor body movements throughout the session, involving both upper and lower extremities and a slow pace (raise the arms, march in place, etc.) for five to 10 minutes until everyone has warmed up.

- Next, invite residents to move their body and extremities following the staff's instructions, gradually increasing the pace. Keep each movement simple and focused on large motor skills. Do this for about 20 minutes.

- A five- to 10-minute period of slower body movements concludes the session. You can use the same movements as those used for the warm-up. Exaggerate the movements so that they are large and slow. You are attempting to relax the residents.

- Thank each participant for joining the group.

- This is a great sensory activity to do in a multisensory room, but if you do not have such a room, make the room as relaxing as possible with subdued lighting and minimal outside distractions.

Variations/adaptations/modifications: You have to adapt/modify your approach based on the physical and cognitive ability level of each individual within the group. Go around and provide the visual, verbal, and direct physical guidance that each person needs to be successful. Redirect as necessary. You will need to offer more assistance to residents with diminished abilities (they may be able to perform tasks with direct hand-over-hand guidance). This requires that you have assessed the abilities and identified the needs, interests, and interventions of each resident in attendance.

Helpful hints/notes: Much of the setup for the activity can be done prior to gathering residents so that you are ready to begin once residents have gathered. Assemble all needed equipment and supplies prior to the start of the activity.

Rice Bag Sensory

Target audience: Residents needing specialized dementia programming and those with behavior issues

Objectives/outcomes:

- To provide tactile stimulation and increase responsiveness

- To provide an opportunity for simple communication

- To promote relaxation, solace, pain management, and enjoyment

- To encourage interaction with others and increase social contact

- To decrease the frequency and severity of symptomatic behavior (tension, anxiety, and agitation)

- To stimulate the senses of withdrawn residents

- To soothe and relax residents who are agitated

- To improve relationships between caregivers and residents

- To help to induce sleep if done in the evening prior to bedtime

Recommended group size: One-on-one in residents' rooms, or in a small group going around one-on-one

Suggested time frame: Approximately five minutes per resident

Special needs/ability level (physical/cognitive skills needed): None

Activity outline:

- You will need rice bags. They are easy to make; simply sew two washcloths together and stuff the resultant bag with rice. To be economical, purchase washcloths in packs of 12 from a discount store (they do not have to be thick washcloths). Get bulk rice from your Dietary Department.

- Always ask for the resident's permission to use the rice bag.

- Heat the bag in a microwave for one minute or less. *Do not* overheat, as there is a potential to burn someone if you do. *Always* test the rice bag on yourself (not on your hands as they can withstand higher temperatures than other places on your skin such as the forearm) for proper temperature. The bag should be warm but not hot. *Do not* place the rice bag directly on the resident's skin. Place it over clothing or have some other material between the rice bag and the resident's bare skin. We recommend that you place the rice bag inside a pillowcase, for two reasons: You can reuse the rice bag because you will not be violating infection control procedures; and the pillowcase provides an extra barrier between the rice bag and the resident's skin.

- If the washcloths become soiled, you will need to remove the rice, wash the washcloths, and refill the bag, or just refill new washcloths that have been sewn together.

- Residents like these placed on their laps when they are in a seated position (their pants or other clothing provides yet another barrier). They are nicely weighted and warm, so residents find them very soothing. They will often place their hands on the bag as well to feel the warmth. We have calmed agitated and anxious residents with this activity.

- This is a great sensory activity to do in a multisensory room, but if you do not have such a room, make the room as relaxing as possible with subdued lighting and minimal outside distractions. Place residents in a circle around the room.

- If you are conducting this activity in a small group setting, play some relaxing background music.

- You can also use an aromatherapy diffuser with a scent that promotes relaxation, such as vanilla or lavender.

Variations/adaptations/modifications: Although this is meant to be a sensory program, alert and oriented residents enjoy it as well. It also can be used to help alleviate pain symptoms. You can also incorporate a therapeutic massage, which is another activity within this chapter.

Helpful hints/notes: You may want to solicit a sewing group to make the rice bags, with you supplying the materials (better yet if the sewing group is willing to supply the materials). Much of the setup for this activity can be done prior to gathering residents so that you are ready to begin once residents have gathered. Assemble all needed equipment and supplies prior to the start of the activity. The facility needs to take measures to ensure resident safety at all times during this activity. You need to have clear directions for the use of the rice bags; the staff needs to know what they are and should be trained in their proper use. There is always a chance that someone will not follow procedure. For example, a few years ago a facility was cited when a staff member put a microwavable item into a microwave for seven minutes and then placed the item around a resident's neck, causing second- and third-degree burns on the resident. As a result, the facility was cited for causing immediate jeopardy to a resident. If the staff member had tested the item to feel how hot it was before placing it on the resident's neck, the incident could have been avoided. We cannot stress enough the importance of having policies in place, and training your staff on the proper use of items within the facility.

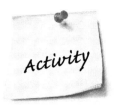
Activity

Rise and Shine

Target audience: Residents needing specialized dementia programming and those with behavioral issues

Objectives/outcomes:

- To provide an opportunity for simple communication

- To provide a pleasurable, failure-free and stress-free environment

- To allow individuals the time, space, and opportunity to enjoy the environment at their own pace, free from unrealistic expectations of others

- To promote large motor physical activity and upper-body range of motion, lower-body movements, communication, and enjoyment

- To encourage interaction with others and increase social contact

- To enhance/increase attention span, thinking and reasoning skills, and concentration, and promote the ability to follow one-step directions or mimic desired actions

- To improve mood by actively engaging residents at their level of ability

- To provide an atmosphere that encourages participants to explore their environment and to be able to enjoy themselves

- To promote the ability of participants to express themselves

- To promote person-centered care

- To improve relationships between caregivers and residents

Recommended group size: Small, or one-on-one

Suggested time frame: 5 – 15 minutes

Special needs/ability level (physical/cognitive skills needed): Residents with the physical capacity to follow one-step directions or mimic desired actions. You need to make sure that residents are able to achieve some level of success in this activity for it to be beneficial to them.

Activity outline:

- This is meant to be an early-morning, first-of-the-day, wake-up-and-get-moving activity.

- Greet each resident by name.

- Verbally state and physically demonstrate each desired action.

- Choose movements that promote the use of large motor skills and have residents repeat each action for five sequences (or whatever level they are able). For example, they can raise their arms straight above their head and lower them; use their arms to make a circle above their head and lower them; put their arms out to the side and bring them together above their head (half of a jumping jack); place their arms out to the side and make small circles, bigger circles, and then really big circles; put their arms out in front of them with their palms facing up and then curl their arms up to touch their shoulders; do wrist circles; make rainfall (by fluttering their fingers); roll their arms (in the same way they would twiddle their thumbs); and perform any other upper-body motion you think they can do. If they are able, have them do some lower-body movements as well (e.g., march in place, lift one knee at a time as high as they can, hold one leg up at a time and do ankle circles, etc.).

- Work with each resident individually as needed, but let them do for themselves as much as they can and provide assistance only if it is truly needed.

- Demonstrate desired actions (visual cues) and provide one-step verbal instructions for each desired action.

- As you are doing the repetitive actions, talk to the residents and provide them with supportive RO (tell them information, rather than grilling them with questions). For example, you can tell them what the weather is, tell them what season it is, tell them of any upcoming events of the day, and so on.

- If you are conducting this activity as a small group, play some lively music to energize the residents, and use aromatherapy of citrus or peppermint.

Variations/adaptations/modifications: You have to adapt/modify your approach based on the physical and cognitive ability level of each individual within the group. Go around and provide the visual, verbal, and direct physical guidance that each person needs to be successful. Redirect as necessary. You will need to offer more assistance to residents with diminished abilities (they may be able to perform tasks with direct hand-over-hand guidance). You may do passive ROM with residents who are unable to do it on their own. This requires that you have assessed the abilities and identified the needs, interests, and interventions of each resident in attendance.

Seashell Sensory

Target audience: Residents needing specialized dementia programming and those with behavior issues

Objectives/outcomes:

- To provide visual, tactile, and auditory stimulation and increase responsiveness

- To provide an opportunity for simple communication

- To promote communication and enjoyment

- To encourage interaction with others and increase social contact

- To enhance/increase attention span, and promote physical movement and reminiscence

- To promote relaxation

- To decrease the frequency and severity of symptomatic behavior (tension, anxiety, and agitation)

- To stimulate the senses of withdrawn residents

- To soothe/relax residents who are agitated

- To improve relationships between caregivers and residents

- To improve mood by actively engaging residents at their level of ability

Recommended group size: Small, or one-on-one

Suggested time frame: 30 minutes

Special needs/ability level (physical/cognitive skills needed): Residents with varying levels of cognitive/physical abilities can join the group, as you work with them individually and provide needed assistance at their ability level. You need to make sure that residents are able to achieve some level of success in this activity for it to be beneficial to them.

Activity outline:

- You will need seashells, white sand, two buckets, and a CD of ocean sounds. It is also nice to have a "wave machine" (an object with liquid inside that moves back and forth, making waves).

- Set up the wave machine and ocean sounds CD (turn up the volume so that it is loud enough for everyone to hear, but soft enough to be relaxing). This is a great sensory activity to do in a multisensory room, but if you do not have such a room, make the room as relaxing as possible with subdued lighting and minimal outside distractions. Place residents in a semi-circle around the room with a view of the wave machine, if you have one.

- Put some seashells in a bucket that residents can see and touch. In the other bucket put the white sand (the sand used in ashtrays works great) and bury some seashells within the sand. Tell the residents to imagine that they are at the seashore and are walking on the beach and gathering seashells. Have each resident take a turn reaching into the sand and removing as many seashells as he or she can find. Make sure every resident who is able gets a chance to participate in this activity as you work your way around the group. You can keep track of who finds the most seashells and make it a challenge game, but you do not need to do this. As you are conducting this activity, prompt discussion with simple, open-ended questions (e.g., Have you ever been to the ocean? Did you ever swim in the ocean? Have you ever gone out to sea? Have you ever walked barefoot along the beach? What did it feel like?).

- You can also use an aromatherapy diffuser with a scent that promotes relaxation, such as vanilla or lavender. Or use an ocean-scented candle with the wick cut off and a candle warmer.

Variations/adaptations/modifications: You could have other seashore items on hand for residents to see and touch (e.g., sea glass devoid of sharp edges, sand dollars, starfish, netting, small lighthouses, etc.). You could have residents match up seashells that are similar instead of just having them see, touch, and find them.

Helpful hints/notes: Much of the setup for this activity can be done prior to gathering residents so that you are ready to begin once residents have gathered. Assemble all needed equipment and supplies prior to the start of the activity.

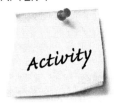

Sensory Stimulation Programs

Target audience: Residents needing specialized dementia programming and those with behavior issues. This activity is designed primarily for residents of very low response who can tolerate being out of bed in a small group setting and who need one-on-one approaches to gain their attention and response.

Objectives/outcomes:

- To offer supportive programs to residents with impaired cognitive and perceptual abilities. These supportive programs will promote resident awareness, responsiveness, and participation (consistent with individual interests, needs, and ability levels).

- To provide visual, tactile, auditory, taste, and olfactory stimulation.

- To provide opportunities for simple communication.

- To encourage residents to follow simple directions.

- To promote remotivation in awareness to the surrounding environment. To provide a pleasurable, failure-free and stress-free environment.

- To allow individuals the time, space, and opportunity to enjoy the environment at their own pace, free from unrealistic expectations of others.

- To promote relaxation, exploration, communication, and enjoyment.

- To encourage interaction with others and increase social contact.

- To decrease the frequency and severity of symptomatic behavior (tension, anxiety, and agitation).

- To stimulate the senses of withdrawn residents.

- To soothe/relax residents who are agitated.

- To enhance/increase attention span, thinking and reasoning skills, memory recall, and concentration.

- To provide opportunities for emotional expression.

- To improve mood by actively engaging residents at their level of ability.

- To provide an atmosphere that encourages participants to explore their environment and to be able to enjoy themselves.

- To promote the ability of participants to express themselves.

- To promote person-centered care.

- To improve relationships between caregivers and residents.

Recommended group size: *One-on-one, or small group

Suggested time frame: 15 – 30 minutes

Special needs/ability level (physical/cognitive skills needed): Residents with varying levels of cognitive/physical abilities can join the group, as you set them up individually with objects at their ability level.

Activity outline:

- Use a portable sensory cart with selected activity materials for varying degrees of cognitive loss (e.g., manipulatives, peg boards, lacing cards, nuts and bolts, PVC piping, music boxes, all-in-one activity boards, color dominoes, simple matching games, sound machines, light-up visuals, themed memory boxes/bags, things to touch, see, and smell, etc.)

- Residents may need to sit at tables for this activity

- Play relaxing background music (auditory) and use aromatherapy, scented beads, and a diffuser, or a candle warmer with a candle (smell)

- Arrange equipment and materials

- Announce the activity and purpose to the residents

- Ask staff members and volunteers to help residents get to and from the activity

- The activity leader should introduce him or herself and use residents' names to help residents maintain or regain some sense of personal orientation

- Present the information in a way that helps to provide supportive RO to residents for increased awareness of the environment

- Introduce and describe the "theme" or items for the day

- Work with each resident individually as needed, but let them do for themselves as much as they can and provide assistance only if it is truly needed

- At the end of the activity thank and praise residents for their participation

Variations/adaptations/modifications: You have to adapt/modify your approach based on the physical and cognitive ability level of each individual within the group. Go around and provide the visual, verbal, and direct physical guidance that each person needs to be successful. Redirect as necessary. You will need to simplify tasks and offer more assistance to residents with diminished abilities (they may be able to perform tasks with direct hand-over-hand guidance).

Helpful hints/notes: *The activities staff and/or trained volunteers may offer sensory stimulation to room-bound or room-preference residents. A hand-held basket or rolling cart can be used to transport materials to the resident's room. Observe all infection-control guidelines and individual resident dietary needs/restrictions when serving food and beverages. Much of the setup for this activity can be done prior to gathering residents so that you are ready to begin once residents have gathered. Assemble all needed equipment and supplies prior to the start of the activity. Clean and disinfect the activity supplies as needed/according to your facility's policy and procedure.

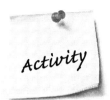

Activity

Sorting Box

Target audience: Residents needing specialized dementia programming and those with behavior issues

Objectives/outcomes:

- To provide visual, tactile, and auditory stimulation and increase responsiveness

- To provide an opportunity for simple communication

- To promote communication and enjoyment

- To encourage interaction with others and increase social contact

- To enhance/increase attention span, concentration, and memory recall, promote physical movement, enhance sorting skills of placing similar objects together, and promote reminiscence

- To promote relaxation

- To decrease the frequency and severity of symptomatic behavior (tension, anxiety, and agitation)

- To stimulate the senses of withdrawn residents

- To soothe/relax residents who are agitated

- To improve relationships between caregivers and residents

- To improve mood by actively engaging residents at their level of ability

Recommended group size: Small, or one-on-one

Suggested time frame: 30 minutes

Special needs/ability level (physical/cognitive skills needed): Residents with varying levels of cognitive/physical abilities can join this group, as you work with them individually and provide needed assistance at their ability level. They need to be able to sort like objects together. You need to make sure that residents are able to achieve some level of success in this activity for it to be beneficial to them.

Activity outline:

- Create various themed sorting boxes—for example, a fishing tackle box into which residents arrange fishing tackle (remove all hooks), a poker chip box into which residents sort poker chips by color (craft boxes with individual compartments work well for this), a sock box into which residents match socks of the same color (use a plastic shoe container for this), large bolts, PVC piping, a greeting card box into which residents sort old greeting cards by theme, a flower box into which residents sort silk flowers by color and/or type (you can provide some unbreakable vases for them to create floral arrangements), and so on

- Work with each resident individually as needed, but let them do for themselves as much as they can and provide assistance only if it is truly needed (you may need to prompt or provide additional clues)

- Keep resident safety in mind, especially in regard to small objects, to prevent residents from placing these objects into their mouths

- You can also use an aromatherapy diffuser with a scent that promotes thinking and concentration, such as citrus or peppermint

Variations/adaptations/modifications: You have to adapt/modify your approach based on the cognitive ability level of each individual. Provide the visual, verbal, and direct physical guidance that each person needs to be successful. Redirect as necessary. You will need to offer more assistance to residents with diminished abilities. This requires that you have assessed the abilities and identified the needs, interests, and interventions of each resident in attendance. This can be an independent activity as long as safety measures are in place (residents are not able to swallow small items). If small items are involved, it's best to work one-on-one with the residents.

Helpful hints/notes: Shop at a dollar store or discount store for items. Clean and disinfect the activity supplies as needed/according to your facility's policy and procedure. Much of the setup for this activity can be done prior to gathering residents so that you are ready to begin once residents have gathered. Assemble all needed equipment and supplies prior to the start of the activity.

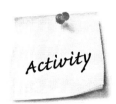

Activity | **Sound Effects Sensory**

Target audience: Residents needing specialized dementia programming and those with behavior issues

Objectives/outcomes:

- To provide visual and auditory stimulation and increase responsiveness

- To provide an opportunity for simple communication

- To promote communication and enjoyment

- To encourage interaction with others and increase social contact

- To enhance/increase attention span, concentration, and memory recall, and promote identification of sounds and reminiscence

- To promote relaxation

- To decrease the frequency and severity of symptomatic behavior (tension, anxiety, and agitation)

- To stimulate the senses of withdrawn residents

- To soothe and relax residents who are agitated

- To improve relationships between caregivers and residents

- To improve mood by actively engaging residents at their level of ability

Recommended group size: Small, or one-on-one

Suggested time frame: 30 minutes

Special needs/ability level (physical/cognitive skills needed): Residents with varying levels of cognitive/physical abilities can join this group, as you work with them individually and provide needed assistance at their ability level. You need to make sure that residents are able to achieve some level of success in this activity for it to be beneficial to them.

Activity outline:

- You will need sound effects CDs and a CD player.

- This is a great sensory activity to do in a multisensory room, but if you do not have such a room, limit outside distractions. Place residents in a circle around the room.

- Explain that you are going to play a variety of sounds and you would like help in identifying what you are hearing. Play one sound at a time and ask the group (or individual) to identify the sound. You may have to replay the sound several times. Once a sound is identified, move on to the next sound. As you are going through the sounds, ask simple, direct (related) questions to promote discussion, thinking, and interaction.

- You can also use an aromatherapy diffuser with a scent that promotes thinking, such as citrus or peppermint.

Variations/adaptations/modifications: You could turn this into a competitive game to see who can identify the most sounds, though this puts pressure on residents to perform, and generally speaking, sensory activities should focus on the experience as a whole and should not pressure residents to perform. You would have to judge the skill level of your residents to determine whether turning this into a competitive game is in their best interests. Some residents with dementia like competition.

Helpful hints/notes: A circle or semi-circle is great for small-group dementia-specific programming, as it promotes eye contact and interaction. You can make your own sound effects tape, but make sure it is of good sound quality; otherwise, residents won't be able to identify the sounds they hear. Generally, these types of CDs are inexpensive and you can easily find them in discount stores, so it usually isn't worth your time and effort to make your own. Much of the setup for this activity can be done prior to gathering residents so that you are ready to begin once residents have gathered. Assemble all needed equipment and supplies prior to the start of the activity.

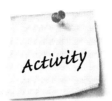

Themed Sensory Kits

Target audience: Residents needing specialized dementia programming and those with behavior issues

Objectives/outcomes:

- To provide visual and tactile stimulation and increase responsiveness

- To provide an opportunity for simple communication

- To promote communication and enjoyment

- To encourage interaction with others and increase social contact

- To enhance/increase attention span and memory recall, and promote physical movement and reminiscence

- To promote relaxation

- To decrease the frequency and severity of symptomatic behavior (tension, anxiety, and agitation)

- To stimulate the senses of withdrawn residents

- To soothe and relax residents who are agitated

- To improve relationships between caregivers and residents

- To improve mood by actively engaging residents at their level of ability

Recommended group size: Small, or one-on-one

Suggested time frame: 30 minutes

Special needs/ability level (physical/cognitive skills needed): Residents with varying levels of cognitive/physical abilities can join this group, as you work with them individually and provide needed assistance at their ability level. This is an especially great activity for residents who like to rummage. You need to make sure that residents are able to achieve some level of success in this activity for it to be beneficial to them.

Activity outline:

- Create various themed kits and place them in boxes/bins or cloth tote bags.

- Here is a list of themed kit topics to get you started: New Year's Day (noisemakers, hats, tiaras, party horns, leis, confetti, etc.); Valentine's Day (red hearts, musical valentine cards, old valentine card covers, heart cookie cutter, cupids, stuffed animals with valentine theme, etc.); St. Patrick's Day (shamrocks, leprechauns, clover cookie cutter, etc.); Easter (plastic Easter eggs that residents can take apart and put together, or you can hide an item inside each egg and have residents try to guess what it is, an Easter basket and bunny, old Easter card covers, etc.); Fourth of July (red, white, and blue as well as patriotic-themed items); Halloween (masks, pumpkins, costumes, etc.); Thanksgiving (cornucopia, recipes for Thanksgiving menu items, fall things); Christmas (old Christmas cards, unbreakable ornaments, garland, small Christmas tree, etc.); baby kit (plastic pants, baby bottle, baby washcloth scented with baby powder or oil, cloth diaper, pacifier, rattle, small doll, baby booties, shoes, and clothing, placed in a diaper bag); sewing/craft kit (old spools of thread, knitting needles, crochet hooks, embroidery hoop, embroidery thread, yarn, and old sewing/craft books, placed in an old sewing box); cooking kit (nesting measuring cups and measuring spoons, wooden spoons, spatula, tongs, baster, apron, pot holder, trivet, recipe cards, etc.); tool kit (level, large bolts, screwdrivers, small wrench, other small tools, tape measure, and ruler, placed in a small toolbox and used only under direct supervision due to safety issues); fishing tackle box (fishing tackle with hooks removed, bobbers, rubber worms and frogs, fishing line etc.); jewelry kit (baubles, beads, lockets, bracelets, pins/brooches, etc., placed in an old time jewelry box); and an old purse (Kleenex, lipstick case, wallet, coin purse, small mirror, embroidered hanky, etc.). Feel free to come up with your own themes for additional kits that participants would enjoy.

- Work with each resident individually as needed, but let them do for themselves as much as they can and provide assistance only if it is truly needed (you may need to prompt or provide additional clues).

- Keep resident safety in mind, especially related to small objects as residents may place them in their mouths.

- You can also use an aromatherapy diffuser with a scent that promotes thinking and concentration, such as citrus or peppermint.

Variations/adaptations/modifications: You have to adapt/modify your approach based on the cognitive ability level of each individual. Provide the visual, verbal, and direct physical guidance that each person needs to be successful. Redirect as necessary. You will need to offer more assistance to residents with diminished abilities. This requires that you have assessed the abilities and identified the needs, interests, and interventions of each resident in attendance. This can be an independent activity as long as safety measures are in place (residents are not able to swallow small items). If small items are involved it's best to work one-on-one with the residents.

Helpful hints/notes: Shop at a dollar store or discount store for items. Go back and shop at every holiday to make holiday-themed kits when in season, as you cannot purchase those items otherwise. Take a cart and go up and down the aisles, creating themed kits as you go for a fraction of the cost. As you go through the aisles other ideas for kits and what to put in them will come to you. You may also want to seek donations from family members, staff members, and volunteers during spring-cleaning time by advertising for needed items that they would probably donate to Goodwill or the church rummage sale, if not to you. Clean and disinfect activity supplies as needed and according to your facility's policy and procedure. Much of the setup for this activity can be done prior to gathering residents so that you are ready to begin once residents have gathered. Assemble all needed equipment and supplies prior to the start of the activity.

Therapeutic Massage

Target audience: Residents needing specialized dementia programming and those with behavior issues

Objectives/outcomes:

- To provide tactile stimulation and increase responsiveness

- To provide an opportunity for simple communication

- To promote relaxation, solace, pain management, and enjoyment

- To encourage interaction with others and increase social contact

- To decrease the frequency and severity of symptomatic behavior (tension, anxiety, and agitation)

- To stimulate the senses of withdrawn residents

- To soothe and relax residents who are agitated

- To improve relationships between caregivers and residents

- To help to induce sleep if done in the evening prior to bedtime

Recommended group size: One-on-one in residents' rooms, or in small groups going around one-on-one

Suggested time frame: Approximately five minutes per resident

Special needs/ability level (physical/cognitive skills needed): None

Activity outline:

- You can use just your hands, or you can also use a wooden bead massager, a soft bristle massage brush, or a battery-operated massager.

- Always ask permission to give a resident a massage. Some people do not like to be touched or to have their personal space invaded.

- Generally speaking, work on the shoulders and upper back and leave neck massages to the true therapists (if giving massages with residents seated in a chair). If you are giving a resident a massage and the resident is lying in bed, you can give a full back massage instead of just the shoulders. Use hand sanitizer between each resident. Because you are not using lotion and are giving the massages over the residents' clothing, you do not have to wash your hands with soap and water between each resident, but you should do so periodically or if you come into contact with a resident's body fluids (e.g., drool).

- If you're using your hands, use a gentle kneading/squeezing action on the upper shoulders and rub gently downward on the resident's arms and down the spine if able. Rub the resident's back as well, asking the resident to lean forward in his or her chair slightly if necessary.

- You can expect to complete six to eight massages in a 30-minute period.

- If you are conducting this activity in a small group setting, play some relaxing background music.

- This is a great sensory activity to do in a multisensory room, but if you do not have such a room, make the room as relaxing as possible with subdued lighting and minimal outside distractions. Place residents in a circle around the room.

Variations/adaptations/modifications: If you're using a massager of some sort, apply only gentle pressure and move the massager in circular motions over the resident's back and shoulders. Wilbarger protocol: helps to reduce verbal and physical aggressive behavior. Using a soft brush, gently and slowly brush down the resident's arms, back, and legs. Repeat several times, while talking in a calm, soothing tone of voice. Then wrap the person in a weighted blanket (weighted blankets are commonly used in sensory rooms, as they provide a pleasant sensation of comfort).

Helpful hints/notes: It is helpful to have a massage therapist demonstrate simple massage techniques that you can perform on your residents. Always keep in mind the fragility of residents' skin and the fact that they can bruise easily. Apply only the amount of pressure that is comfortable and appropriate for them.

Chapter 5

Adapting and Modifying Activities to Accommodate Individual Resident Needs

The ultimate goals of any activity are to provide enjoyment, and to be engaging and meaningful to the participant(s). This often requires making adaptations to meet the specific needs of individual residents, thereby providing them with some measure of success. If an activity is frustrating to residents because it requires skill that is beyond their abilities, this defeats the whole purpose of providing the activity.

In its revised activities guidance to surveyors, the Centers for Medicare & Medicaid Services (CMS) has identified the process of making adaptations as an important role of activities professionals. CMS mandates that facilities make efforts to provide needed adaptations and assistance to enable residents to pursue their leisure interests. This means assessing and planning the care for each resident to identify any limitations and specific adaptations that are needed to address conditions and issues affecting the resident's participation in activities. Facilities need to provide any necessary supplies and adaptive equipment to individual residents to optimize and facilitate their participation.

Adaptations also apply to other staff members who provide care and activities to residents. All staff members who provide activities to residents need to be able to offer adaptive assistance to residents who need it, and they must be familiar with the proper use of the equipment according to each resident's care plan. This includes making adaptations to the activity, the environment, and the situation. Residents may have limitations due to various social/communication, cognitive, or physical impairments. Some adaptations include special equipment and special techniques, and others involve adapting the environment where the activities are taking place.

Many activities can be adapted to accommodate a particular resident's change in functioning. Facilities should be aware of the range of adaptations they can make to assist residents in participating in activities of their choice. Many different adaptations can be used for the various impairments that residents may have. The following chart identifies some common impairments that require adaptations, and effective interventions for each.

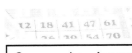

Common Impairments and Adaptations/Interventions

Common Impairments	Adaptations/Interventions
Many things can contribute to the need for environmental modifications. They include: • Visual impairments • Hearing impairments • Physical impairments • Cognitive impairments • Communication barriers • Mobility impairments	**Environmental Modifications** • Eliminate glare • Provide appropriate/better lighting • Control temperature • Reduce extraneous noise • Ensure that table heights accommodate wheelchair users • Have all supplies within the reach of residents • Secure supplies • Eliminate excess activity and distractions
Physical Limitations: • Loss of upper/lower-extremity function • Limited ROM • Loss of hand dexterity • Hemiplegic	• Provide proper seating and positioning • Place supplies and materials within easy access • Offer larger handles or built-up equipment • Provide holders (e.g., book holder, C-clamp, suction vise, rubber mat/dycem to secure items in place, card shuffler, adapted tools) • Move targets closer (for recreational games) and make needed compensations • Provide verbal and visual cues • Offer hand-over-hand guidance/direct physical guidance • Simplify tasks • Provide voice activity computer • Provide page turners • Provide mouth pieces • Slow down the action or activity • Offer exercises and activities to build strength and endurance
Cognitive Limitations: • Impaired ability to follow directions • Impaired ability to comprehend/language • Impaired ability to process information/processing speed • Impaired thinking/reasoning skills • Impaired hand-eye coordination • Impaired verbal skills • Impaired ability to learn • Impaired ability to plan and carry out tasks	• Segment and simplify tasks • Target programs using retained long-term memory • Alter length of program based on attention span • Redirect resident to task/activity at hand • Provide one-step directions • Demonstrate desired action • Use gestures

5

ADAPTING AND MODIFYING ACTIVITIES TO ACCOMMODATE INDIVIDUAL RESIDENT NEEDS

THE BIG BOOK OF RESIDENT ACTIVITIES

225

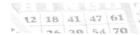

Common Impairments and Adaptations/Interventions (cont.)	
• Impaired ability to follow verbal and visual cues • Limited attention span • Forgetfulness • Disorientation/memory loss • Repetitive behaviors • Impaired ability to concentrate • Impaired memory recall • Decreased responses to stimulation/ environment • Decreased physical movement • Increased anxiousness/agitation • Decreased awareness of the environment • Decreased social displays • Decreased comfort levels	• Provide additional verbal and visual cues • Repeat as necessary • Provide hand-over-hand guidance/direct physical guidance • Target past experiences/interests • Increase stimulation • Decrease stimulation • Offer small groups with no interruptions/ distractions • Use prompts and props • Provide a set routine • Be flexible in your approach • Validate residents' feelings • Provide constant direction and supervision • Build on any retained abilities no matter how small • Use concrete phrases • Speak slowly and distinctly • Allow adequate time for residents to understand and give a response • Offer simple choices, but limit choices • Provide praise and reassurance • Remind and repeat gently • Ask only one question at a time • Provide task-oriented activities • Provide stimulation to the environment • Provide sorting activities • Provide short, structured activities that focus on simple tasks • (See Chapter 4 for additional information.)
Language/Communication Limitations: • Impaired processing of information • Impaired ability to understand • Impaired speech • Unfamiliar language	• Allow adequate time for processing information and formulating response • Use communication boards • Use translation tools • Use audio/visual materials • Utilize staff members who speak the resident's primary language • Have an interpreter on call • Use family assistance in communicating with the resident (See also adaptations for cognitive limitations.)

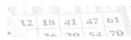

Common Impairments and Adaptations/Interventions (cont.)

Mobility Limitations: • Inability to walk unassisted • Limited use of upper or lower extremities • Hemiplegic	• Provide needed assistive devices (e.g., walker, cane, wheelchair) • Walk with the resident • Provide assistance in transportation to and from activities • Provide closer targets and make needed compensations • Have resident use his or her unaffected side • Provide exercises and activities to build strength and endurance
Visual Limitations: • Impaired/poor eyesight • Blindness • Visual field neglect • Brightness hurts eyes	• Increase the lighting level without creating glare • Ensure that residents' eyeglasses are clean and that the prescription is correct • Provide magnifying glasses • Provide light-filtering lenses • Provide telescopic lenses • Use the clock method of identification • Describe size, shape, color, placement, etc. • Offer large-print reading material, cards, and books • Provide audio books • Keep things in the same place in the resident's room • Provide verbal cues • Offer direct physical guidance • Provide hand-over-hand guidance • Place objects on the resident's unaffected side, in his or her field of vision • Remind residents to turn or look to their affected side • Provide small-group activities • Place residents near the activity • Have a staff member or volunteer assist • Use contrasting colors, bold type/print
Hearing Limitations: • Impaired/poor hearing • Deafness	• Have residents wear dark glasses • Provide personal hearing aides • Provide hearing devices (headphones, amplifiers) • Offer closed-captioning TV • Decrease background noise • Provide written instructions

Common Impairments and Adaptations/Interventions (cont.)

	• Use gestures/sign language • Utilize props and pictures • Use translation tools/communication tools (e.g., picture charts/communication boards/visual tools) • Place residents near the sound source of the activity • Have a staff member or volunteer assist • Attract the resident's attention and establish eye contact • Face the person and get at his or her eye level • Speak slowly and distinctly • Repeat or rephrase statements or questions • Ask only one question at a time • Use a microphone

Chapter 6

Activities for Younger Residents and Short-Term Stay Residents

As a result of the "aging in place" and "least restrictive environment" trends, long-term care facilities are seeing more admissions for short-term rehab stay residents versus long-term care residents. The aforementioned trends relate to keeping people in their homes for as long as possible, and to discharging residents from long-term care facilities to an environment that meets their needs/level of care and that is least restrictive (and generally less costly). Often, a facility's younger residents are also short-term stay residents.

Both younger and short-term residents can present unique challenges to the activities professional, as they generally have a different set of needs, preferences, and leisure interests. The mandate of the Centers for Medicare & Medicaid Services to provide an ongoing program of activities designed to meet, in accordance with the comprehensive assessment, the interests and the physical, mental, and psychosocial well-being of each resident dictates that facilities accommodate the leisure pursuits of short-term residents. And therein lies the challenge. These residents are not your "typical" elderly residents who can "fit" into your established program based on your long-term residents' needs, preferences, and leisure interests. Therefore, to accommodate the specific needs of short-term stay and younger residents, you must start by conducting a comprehensive assessment and care plan. Then you must offer different activities based on these residents' needs and preferences.

Younger residents usually have very different preferences related to their activity pursuits compared to those of long-term residents. After all, they come from a whole different generation. For example, many prefer independent in-room activities. They do not see themselves as joining in groups with the "elderly." In addition, many are "baby boomers." They tend to expect service, privacy, independence, and choice, and they expect that things will be done their way. They want to "age in place" and not reside in long-term living situations outside a rehab stay.

The main focus or goal of most short-term rehab stay residents is rehabilitation to the point where they regain their independence and can return to their former living situation, or at least can be in a facility that is more home-like and less restrictive to them.

Activities professionals need to recognize these residents' goals and preferences and develop an individualized activity plan of care that is specific to each resident (as they do for all residents). This may mean bringing the activity to them, providing activities and supplies in their room that they can pursue in their own time, and helping them to self-structure their own day. If they are able to independently pursue their own activities, this should be noted in their assessment. If a resident has a preference for independent activities and/or in-room activities, the staff should note whether there is anything they need to do repeatedly to help the resident obtain the necessary supplies. The staff also needs to make sure each resident is informed about activities in the facility, and should periodically ask residents whether they wish to attend anything. In addition, the staff should determine whether a resident's present pattern of leisure pursuits is a lifelong pattern and whether the resident is content with his or her choice. Remember, residents are not required to attend activities. However, some residents may change their minds as they become familiar with the facility and with other residents (i.e., they make friends), and as they establish a rapport with the staff. It's all about meeting the individual needs, preferences, and desires of the residents.

Another consideration for activities professionals is that these residents are most often involved extensively in therapy. In fact, they are often in therapy for much of the morning and afternoon; hence, they are often tired and need to rest in between therapy sessions. As such, they tend to pursue leisure interests in the evenings or when they are not involved in therapy or are resting; therefore, they may have limited energy, time, and, often, desire for leisure pursuits. Leisure pursuits may have to be at the low-energy level.

Activities professionals should work with the therapy department to help residents reach their therapy goals when possible. This means providing activities that complement therapies and that help them to regain their strength, endurance, and independence so that they can be discharged to their previous living situation or to a less-restrictive environment. Offering various forms of exercise is an example. Younger residents may enjoy tai chi, yoga, Pilates, martial arts, and a walking club (they may be a "mall walker" and walking halls with other short-term stay residents would be similar in nature).

Other activities to offer to younger residents and short-term stay residents include computer and Internet access; daily crosswords, word searches, and trivia games (have these on hand in the therapy department or in a place where they can pick them up in their daily travels); a daily trivia board situated where they can see it while on their way to and from therapy; an in-room weekend trivia game; having them assist with facility mailings (this helps with occupational therapy goals); social gatherings for just the younger and/or short-term stay residents; and a welcoming or guardian program. A facility can also provide a travel cart (for in-room activities) equipped with a TV and VCR/DVD player and tapes/DVDs, a Wii game console (or something similar), handheld games, card and board games, a CD player and a variety of CDs, and so on. It is also appropriate to encourage family members to bring in any leisure supplies that are specific to their loved one to allow the resident to self-structure his or her day as he or she would at home (e.g., a personal collection of music, videos, DVDs, craft supplies, etc.).

You can use any of the following activities to enhance programming for short-term rehab stay residents and younger residents. (These are also good activities for long-term stay residents as well.)

Daily Crossword or Trivia

Target audience: Younger residents and short-term stay rehab residents

Objectives/outcomes:

- To provide and promote meaningful leisure pursuits

- To stimulate mental functioning

- To promote independence in structuring day

Recommended group size: Independent, in-room

Suggested time frame: Not applicable

Special needs/ability level (physical/cognitive skills needed): Ability to read and write, cognitive skills, thinking skills, ability to pursue leisure interests independently

Activity outline:

- Find a resource for crosswords or trivia. Resources include books (which you can buy at Wal-Mart and at dollar discount stores) and the Internet. One Internet site to use is *www.dellmagazines.com/*.

- Run off a predetermined number of copies (enough for those who want to take part; you will come to know this through trial and error).

- Place the puzzles in a flat office letterbox labeled "Daily Crossword/Trivia" and leave it in the activity area; you could place another box in the therapy department and/or on the Medicare unit. The idea is to promote residents' independence and to have them take the initiative to come and get the puzzle daily. (If a resident is interested but is physically unable to get his or her own copy, of course the staff should take it to the resident's room.)

- Post the answer page the following day in a predetermined area(s).

- Provide this activity daily, or Monday through Thursday. (See "Weekend Trivia" for an idea for Friday.)

Variations/adaptations/modifications: Residents who are blind or have limited vision can have staff members, volunteers, or family members read the trivia questions to them and they can provide the answers. You could also pair up roommates/peers to assist one another. Residents can work on them as a group when they are together in therapy, or when they are sitting together at meal time. Residents who like to use the computer can go online and get their own puzzles. You could also create a daily trivia board (displayed in a high-traffic area where residents can see it daily). There you can post a daily trivia question and then post the answer and a new question the next day. You could turn this into a contest and have residents submit their answers in writing in a special mailbox, and then hold a monthly drawing in which you select a winner from all the residents who answered all the questions correctly. Open the contest to residents, family members, volunteers, and all staff members. This activity promotes daily discussion among the staff, family members, volunteers, and residents. You may be surprised at how popular this activity can be.

Helpful hints/notes: Advertise and promote this activity during groups, during activity assessments, during resident council meetings and other meetings, within your activities schedule of events, and/or in your facility newsletter. Remember to observe all copyright laws.

Library Cart

Target audience: Younger residents and short-term stay rehab residents

Objectives/outcomes:

- To provide and promote meaningful leisure pursuits

- To stimulate mental functioning

- To promote independence in structuring day

Recommended group size: Independent, in-room

Suggested time frame: As needed for volunteers to complete the room-to-room visits

Special needs/ability level (physical/cognitive skills needed): Ability to read, cognitive skills, thinking skills, ability to pursue leisure interests independently

Activity outline:

- Have the local library provide you with reading materials, both regular and large print, in a variety of topics to meet the expressed interests of your residents (e.g., fiction, nonfiction, romance, mystery, biography, etc.). Routinely rotate the materials on a scheduled basis.

- Subscribe to or seek donations of various magazines of interest to your residents.

- Set up a volunteer to conduct library cart visits. The cart should be stocked with books and magazines.

- Have a checkout system in place for safe return of reading materials for others' future use.

- Allow residents to peruse reading materials and make their selections.

- Encourage volunteers to also make this a social visit.

- Routinely recycle old magazines to keep magazine offerings current.

- Provide this activity on a weekly basis.

Variations/adaptations/modifications: Residents who are blind or have limited vision can have a staff member, volunteer, or family member read to them, or you can have books on tape available for them. You could also pair up roommates/peers to assist one another. Keep a supply of donated books and magazines in the lounge areas as well for easy access.

Helpful hints/notes: Advertise and promote this activity during groups, during activity assessments, during resident council meetings and other meetings, within your activities schedule of events, and/or in your facility newsletter.

Martial Arts/Adapted Tae Kwon Do

Target audience: Younger residents and short-term stay rehab residents

Objectives/outcomes:

- To build staff and resident rapport

- To help build relationships among residents with similar interests and abilities

- To provide an opportunity for socialization

- To enhance therapy goals

- To promote a healthy lifestyle

- To improve balance and reduce the risk of falls

- To improve mobility and function

- To improve coordination

- To improve cardiovascular endurance

- To improve mind-body coordination

- To decrease joint pain

- To improve blood pressure and circulation

- To decrease depression

- To improve cognition and short-term memory

- To enhance vitality and energy

- To build strength and endurance and help residents regain their independence

Recommended group size: Can vary, but should be manageable to the leader

Suggested time frame: 30 – 45 minutes

Special needs/ability level (physical/cognitive skills needed): Individuals who can follow actions and physically complete a series of movements

Activity outline:

- Tae kwon do (a Korean form of martial arts) mostly involves kicking while moving the hands and arms to simulate punches and blocks. Warming up and stretching is extremely important to avoid injuries. Participants should not complete any sequence that causes pain. Inform participants to do the exercises at a slow pace to the best of their ability, and to rest when they need to. Tell participants that if they experience pain they should not perform that movement. All of the movements described in this activity are adapted for a seated position. All movements are meant to be repeated. Movements in tae kwon do are completed in a series of 10 and are counted aloud in Korean. Residents may find it interesting to learn to count to 10 in Korean (hana, dool, tset, net, da-sut, yeo-sut, il-gop, yeo-dul, ah-hop, and yeol). For pronunciation, *d* sounds like *t* in *dool*; in *tset* the *t* is silent; *da-sut* is pronounced *da-sit*; the *o* is silent in *yeo-sut*, so yeo-sut rhymes with da-sut; the *p* is silent in *il-gop*; *yeo-dul* is pronounced *yaalldul*; and *yeol* is pronounced *yea all*.

- Start with martial arts warm-up exercises. Have participants do movements slowly and deliberately and hold stretches before repeating a sequence. Follow this sequence:

  – Begin by placing your arms out to your sides. Raise your arms above your head while inhaling deeply, then slowly lower your arms back to your sides as you exhale. Repeat several times.

  – Do modified jumping jacks (complete the motion with just the upper body/arms).

  – Lean to the left, right, and forward, rotate your arms forward and then backward, tilt your head to the left, back, right, and forward, and then do slow neck rotations.

  – Place your hands on your hips and do slow body trunk rotations, first to the left and then to the right.

  – Place your hands on your knees and do slow knee rotations, first to the left and then to the right.

  – Grasp your wrist and gently stretch your arm forward, then cross your arm over to the side and place your other arm between your elbow and shoulder to gently stretch the arm. Repeat on the other side.

- Bend forward and reach as far to the floor as you safely can. Repeat several times.

- Reach to left and then to the right as far as you safely can. Repeat several times.

- Raise your left leg and hold; repeat several times. Then raise your right leg and hold; repeat several times.

- Do front kicks, alternating sides.

- Raise your legs and hold them in the air, and do a lower-extremity jumping jack motion.

- End by rotating your ankles, first one leg and then the other.

• The following are some additional moves based on tae kwon do movements:

- Have your guard up (arms protecting your chest and hands in fists). With your left hand above your right hand, jab (punch outward with your left hand and bring it back) and cross (punch outward with your right hand and bring it back). (Jabs are done with the leading or upper hand and crosses are done with the other hand.) Repeat these movements several times.

- Switch positions so that your right hand is above your left hand, and then jab and cross. Repeat these movements several times.

- Combine these movements with kicks by jabbing, crossing, and then kicking with the leg/foot of the same side that did the jab. Repeat several times and then switch hand positions and do the same sequence of movements. (You can also do jab, cross, upper cut (as though you are going to punch someone under the chin), and jab, cross, side punch (as though you are going to punch someone on the side of his or her head).

• Here are some block movements residents can do:

- Down block: Put your left arm straight down to the knee and your right hand in a fist on your right hip. Switch by bringing your right arm up to your left shoulder and simultaneously lowering your right arm straight down to your right knee and bringing your left hand up into a fist on your left hip. Reverse and repeat this motion back and forth.

- High or upper block: Begin with your left arm curved above your head in a fist and your right hand in a fist on your right hip. As you lower your left arm in front of you, bring your right arm up in front and over your left arm (so that they cross at chest level). Continue bringing your right arm up above your head in a fist and your left arm down to your left hip in a fist. Reverse and repeat this motion back and forth.

– Inner block: Bend your left arm over your chest near your right shoulder, make a fist, place your right arm on your right hip, and make a fist. Bring your right arm up to your ear and switch/swing your right arm over your chest near your left shoulder in a fist and your left arm in a fist on your left hip. Reverse and repeat this motion back and forth.

– Outer block: Bend your left arm up and make a fist, and place your right fist on your right hip. Reach over to your left side with your right arm as though you are grabbing something and pulling it back to your right, but as you pull back raise your right arm into a bent position and in a fist and place your left fist on your left hip. Reverse and repeat this motion back and forth.

– Knife hand block: Cup both hands. Put your left hand in front so that you can see over it and your right hand on your navel. Swing your arms up and to the left; as you bring them back, place your right arm out in front and your left hand over your navel. Reverse and repeat several times.

– Spear hand block: Cup both hands. Extend your left arm out in front, resting on top of your right hand. Bend your left arm at the elbow and bring it over to your right elbow. Pull your right arm back and shoot it straight out in front of you over your left hand. Reverse and repeat several times.

– Sword hand block: Bend your left arm at the elbow and put it out in front of you. Have your hand in an open knife position as though you struck someone in the side of his or her neck. Make a fist with your right hand and put it on your right hip. Bring your right arm up to your ear with your hand in an open knife position. Simultaneously bring your left arm back to your left hip in a fist position and sweep your right arm/hand to the left as though you are hitting someone in the neck. Reverse and repeat several times.

• If you have more capable residents who can do tae kwon do moves from a standing position, a good resource is *The State of the Art: Taekwondo* (Broadway, 1999). This book explains and shows tae kwon do basics including blocks, stances, punches, kicks, and forms.

Variations/adaptations/modifications: Residents who sit in wheelchairs can perform these actions from a sitting position with the leader's help. You will need to know the individual abilities of each resident and provide the needed modifications. Provide verbal and visual cues. Simplify movements as needed.

Helpful hints/notes: Advertise and promote this activity during groups, during activity assessments, during resident council meetings and at other meetings, through your therapy department, within your activities schedule of events, and/or in your facility newsletter. Consult a doctor to ensure safety for each participant. Make sure the floor is not slippery. Have participants wear comfortable shoes and clothing. Make sure participants drink plenty of water and take frequent breaks. Invite a martial arts instructor for demonstrations and advice on setting up a safe and effective program for participants.

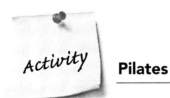

Activity

Pilates

Target audience: Younger residents and short-term stay rehab residents

Objectives/outcomes:

- To build staff and resident rapport

- To help build relationships among residents with similar interests and abilities

- To provide an opportunity for socialization

- To enhance therapy goals

- To promote a healthy lifestyle

- To improve balance and reduce the risk of falls

- To improve mobility and function

- To improve coordination

- To improve cardiovascular endurance

- To improve mind-body coordination

- To decrease joint pain

- To promote relaxation

- To alleviate chronic pain

- To improve sleep

- To reduce stiffness

- To help prevent sarcopenia (progressive muscle loss)

- To help prevent bone loss

- To improve blood pressure and circulation

- To decrease depression

- To improve cognition and short-term memory

- To enhance vitality and energy

- To build strength and endurance and help residents regain their independence

Recommended group size: Can vary, but should be manageable to the leader

Suggested time frame: 30 – 45 minutes

Special needs/ability level (physical/cognitive skills needed): Individuals who can follow actions and physically complete a series of movements

Activity outline:

- Pilates involves working the core muscles, which protects the lower back, develops strength, and lengthens muscles. It's a method of complete mental and physical conditioning. By practicing the movements you become more aware of your body. Movements can be small and therapeutic (designed to help people recover from injuries) or intensified to be more challenging. There are 34 original Pilates movements. Pilates involves concentration, breathing, centering, control, precision, movement, isolation, and routine. All movements in these exercises should involve smooth, continuous motion. Abdominals should be engaged for each movement as well.

- Begin by practicing the breathing technique. Pull your navel to your spine and up to your rib cage. Breathe into your lower rib cage. You should feel and see your ribs expand. Practice this breathing technique.

- For warm-ups, sit quietly with your feet flat on the floor and your arms down at your sides. Rock your heels and toes back and forth, keeping your abdominals engaged. Now roll your shoulders back. Stretch as though someone is lifting your head to the ceiling. Continue practicing breathing into your ribs, not your abdominals. Relax.

- With your arms down at your sides, inhale while reaching through your fingertips and up to shoulder height. Exhale, and continue up above your head. Inhale, and lower your arms/hands to your sides. Repeat this sequence several times.

- With your arms out in front, inhale and bring one arm up and the other down. Exhale and alternate your arms with your breaths.

- Hold your arms out in front with your hands cupped together. Inhale and open and raise your arms (making a V shape), exhale, and bring your arms back down together in front of you. Repeat this sequence several times. Bring your arms back to rest at your sides.

- Sit straight, with your feet flat on the floor and your knees together. Inhale, raise your knees by rocking up on your toes, and bring your arms down to your sides. Exhale, put your heels down on the floor, and raise your arms above your head. Repeat this sequence several times.

- With your arms at your sides, alternate your arms by making floating circles from front to back and left to right. Inhale as you bring your arms up and exhale as you bring them back and down.

- Sit straight, with your feet flat on the floor and your abs engaged. With your arms hanging down at your sides, do shoulder circles back and down. Inhale as you bring your shoulders up and exhale as you bring them down.

- With your feet flat on the floor and your hands on your thighs, breathe out and round out your back as you lean forward. Breathe in as you return. Repeat several times.

- Stretch your arms up to the ceiling as you breathe in. Breathe out and swing your arms down and back, bending forward. Breathe in and bring your arms and body back up. Repeat in a fluid motion several times.

- With your arms hanging at your sides, breathe out and slowly roll forward and down one vertebra at a time. Breathe in and slowly roll back up. Repeat.

- The next four sequences use a resistance band. Hold the resistance band with both hands out in front of you. Inhale, and raise your hands to your shoulder; exhale, and raise your hands up above your head. Inhale, and lower your hands to your shoulder; exhale, taking your hands all the way down. Repeat this sequence several times.

- To stretch your chest, place a resistance band behind and around your back, holding one end in each hand. With your arms extended in front of you, breathe out and reach your arms up and out to your sides. Breathe in and close your arms (make a V shape). Repeat this sequence several times.

- To twist your spine, breathe in and extend your arms out to your sides; breathe out and turn to your right, and breathe in and bring your arms back to the center. With your arms extended, breathe out and turn to the left. Continue this sequence several times.

- With your arms down in front of you and one end of the band in each hand, inhale and bring your arms up; exhale and lean to the left. Inhale and come back up to the center, and then exhale and bring your arms back down in front of you. Inhale and bring your arms up, exhale and lean to the right; inhale and come back up to the center, then exhale and bring your arms back down in front of you. Repeat this sequence several times. Put the resistance bands down.

- With your hands on your thighs, inhale and roll your body down, with your hands going down your legs. Inhale and roll back up, stretching through your spine. Repeat this sequence several times.

- Sit with your feet flat on the floor. Inhale and bring your left knee up, and exhale and extend your leg. Inhale and bring your leg back. Exhale and place your leg down. Inhale and bring your right knee up, and exhale and extend your leg. Inhale and bring your leg back, exhale and place your leg down. Repeat several sequences.

- Inhale and lift your left leg as high as you can, exhale, and lower it back to the floor. Inhale and lift your right leg as high as you can, exhale, and lower it back to the floor. Repeat this sequence several times.

- As though you are swimming, alternate left leg kicks with right leg kicks, raising your legs about 6 inches from the floor. Do 10 for each leg, or 20 kicks total. Now bring in arm movements as well. As your left leg comes up, your right arm comes up; as your right leg comes up, your left arm comes up. Inhale and exhale on the up and down motions. Repeat several sequences.

- In a sitting position, with your feet crossed at the ankles, pull your navel back and up. Breathe into your rib cage and roll your shoulders back, lengthening the neck. Lift your arms to your sides, shoulder height. Bring your arms to the front and cross them over your chest. Inhale and turn/twist to the left, exhale and come back to the center. Inhale and turn/twist to the right, exhale and come back to the center. Continue with a smooth, continuous motion for several sequences.

- Come back to the center, exhale, bring your arms down, and relax.

Variations/adaptations/modifications: Residents who sit in wheelchairs can perform these actions from a sitting position with a leader's help. You will need to know the individual abilities of each resident and provide the needed modifications. Provide verbal and visual cues. Simplify movements as needed.

Helpful hints/notes: Advertise and promote this activity during groups, during activity assessments, during resident council meetings and at other meetings, through your therapy department, within your activities schedule of events, and/or in your facility newsletter. Consult a doctor to ensure safety for each participant. Make sure the floor is not slippery. Have participants wear comfortable shoes and clothing. Make sure participants drink plenty of water and take frequent breaks.

Social Time

Target audience: Younger residents and short-term stay rehab residents

Objectives/outcomes:

- To provide and promote meaningful leisure pursuits

- To provide socialization opportunities

- To provide opportunities to form friendships with others with similar interests and abilities

- To provide a comfortable, nonthreatening environment for the enjoyment of socialization

Recommended group size: Can vary from small to large

Suggested time frame: 45 – 60 minutes

Special needs/ability level (physical/cognitive skills needed): Individuals with varying physical and cognitive skills can participate in this activity.

Activity outline:

- Purchase all needed supplies and keep them on hand: beer (both alcoholic and non-alcoholic), brandy (flavored if desired), whiskey, vodka, mixers, wine, and soda (for those desiring nonalcoholic choices).

- Have a predetermined "menu" of options (e.g., Old-Fashioned, sour, and sweet with brandy or whiskey, Bloody Marys, beer, wine, and soda).

- Have a "waitress" go table to table and take drink orders.

- Have a "bartender" mix the drinks.

- Have other staff members or volunteers serve the drinks as they are made.

- Serve a snack as well (pretzels, cheese curls, cheese and crackers, popcorn, etc.).

- Play background music of the residents' choosing, or have a musician play background music. You don't want the music to be overbearing, as you want residents to socialize with others at their tables.

Variations/adaptations/modifications: For a large group, all residents can be included. You could provide this to a smaller group for just younger and/or short-term rehab residents. You can do different variations (e.g., a Grasshopper Social, a Margarita Social, etc., by offering specialty drinks instead of an open bar).

Helpful hints/notes: Observe all infection-control guidelines and individual resident dietary needs/restrictions when serving food and beverages. You must know of any food allergies your residents may have. Do not include residents who have a known alcohol addiction, who have a contraindication, or are not of legal drinking age. You should have policies and procedures in place for this activity (how much alcohol per drink, how many drinks allowed per resident, the need for a doctor's order, etc.). Much of the setup for this event can be done prior to gathering residents so that you are ready to begin once residents have gathered. Assemble all needed equipment and supplies prior to the start of the activity.

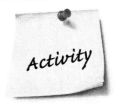

Tai Chi

Target audience: Younger residents and short-term stay rehab residents

Objectives/outcomes:

- To build staff and resident rapport

- To help build relationships among residents with similar interests and abilities

- To provide an opportunity for socialization

- To enhance therapy goals

- To promote a healthy lifestyle

- To improve balance and reduce the risk of falls

- To improve mobility and function

- To improve coordination

- To improve cardiovascular endurance

- To improve mind-body coordination

- To decrease joint pain

- To promote relaxation

- To alleviate chronic pain

- To improve sleep

- To reduce stiffness

- To help prevent sarcopenia (progressive muscle loss)

- To help prevent bone loss

- To improve blood pressure and circulation

- To decrease depression

- To improve cognition and short-term memory

- To enhance vitality and energy

- To build strength and endurance and helps residents regain their independence

Recommended group size: Can vary, but should be manageable to the leader

Suggested time frame: 30 – 45 minutes

Special needs/ability level (physical/cognitive skills needed): Individuals who can follow actions and physically complete a series of movements

Activity outline:

- Tai chi involves slow, graceful, dance-like movements, which are safe for all to perform at any age.

- As always, for any exercise, begin with a brief warm-up and gentle stretching exercises. Begin by standing or sitting with your feet flat on the floor, with your arms hanging down at your sides and your hands in fists. Open your hands slowly while relaxing your shoulders. Focus on the palms of your hands, breathing slowly and deeply while relaxing your stomach. While breathing in, slowly lift your arms to the side, parallel to the floor. While breathing out, slowly lower your arms to the initial position. While breathing in, raise one leg, and while breathing out lower your leg back to the floor. Repeat with the other leg.

- Here are some simple tai chi moves:

  - Front static stance: Hold your head upright, shoulders relaxed, chest relaxed, wrists and fingers extended, and elbows slightly flared. Your hips are expanded, knees are slightly bent, and feet are slightly more than shoulder-width apart.

  - Bellowing inhale: Breathe in through your nose until your whole body is filled with air as you bring your arms up and out to the side, palms up. Do not force it.

  - Bellowing exhale: Breath out through your nose normally. As you breathe out, imagine the whole universe condensing into your lower abdomen. Bend forward at the waist and clasp your wrists down in front.

  - Bear swing: Bend your arms in front of you, twist your waist to the right side, and then twist your waist to the left side. This is called a "bear swing" because it resembles a bear scratching its back on a tree. (If you're standing, your legs should be front on 1.5 times shoulder width, and you should shift your weight from one leg to the other as you twist from side to side, with your arms down while imagining you are holding a 10-pound bag of rice and moving it from side to side.)

- Roll back: Hold your hands out in front of you, palms up, and with arms bent at the elbows. Push forward as you lean forward. Rock back into the original position and repeat. (If you're standing, stand with one leg in front of the other and shift your weight back and forth as you move back and forth.) Put your arms out in front of you, palms up and arms bent at the elbows, swing arms and hands to the left side and up slightly. Bring back to front position and swing hands to right side and up slightly. Repeat back and forth.

- Silk reeling: Put your left arm straight out in front, palm up, and grasp your left wrist with your right hand. Slowly make large circles with your right hand. Reverse to the other side.

- Threading: Put your right arm straight out in front of you with your right palm up, and your left arm bent at the elbow and your left palm up and resting on the inside elbow of your right arm. Swing your left arm straight out and your right arm over so that your hand rests on the inside elbow of your left arm, palm up. Repeat back and forth.

- Encircle the moon: With your body slightly turned to the left, put your right hand in front of your face and your left hand down on your side, and lean your body back slightly. Turn your body slightly to the right, and bring your right hand to the side in a "shielding" action while bringing your left hand in front of your face, also in a shielding action.

- Rolling, grinding ball: Stand with your left hand in front of your chest, your palm facing down, and your right hand with your palm up slightly below your navel. Imagine holding a big ball in front of your chest. Slowly rotate the ball counter-clockwise until the right hand is on the top, the left hand is on the bottom, and the palms are facing each other. Now rotate the ball clockwise. Repeat this motion back and forth several times.

• You may want to try using a weighted tai chi ball. Here are three exercises to try with a tai chi ball:

- With your arms down on both sides and the ball in one hand, slowly raise your arms from the sides, bend them over your head, and slowly move your hands down past your chest toward your stomach. Once your hands are below your stomach, switch the ball to the other hand and repeat the process. Remember to keep your body relaxed at all times. Inhale when lifting your arms and exhale when lowering them. Repeat the process at least five times.

- Place both hands beneath your stomach, with the ball in one hand and your palms facing up. Slowly raise both hands toward the front of your chest. Continue lifting your arms toward the sky. Make sure your palms are facing up (hold for a moment and look up). Allow both arms to slowly glide down your sides, switching the ball to the other hand once at the bottom. Repeat at least five times. Your head and neck should be relaxed at all times. Remember to inhale when lifting your arms and to exhale when lowering them.

- Raise both arms toward the front of your chest, palms facing up. Lift your right arm, palm facing up (holding the ball) toward the sky. At the same time, lower your left arm, palm facing down toward the ground. Hold this position and stretch for a few minutes. Slowly glide both arms back into the original position in front of your chest and switch the ball to the other hand; follow through the process on the opposite side. Repeat at least five times. Exhale when your arms are stretching and inhale when they are at chest level.

Variations/adaptations/modifications: Residents who sit in wheelchairs can perform these actions from a sitting position with help from the leader. You will need to know the individual abilities of each resident and provide the needed modifications. Provide verbal and visual cues. Simplify movements as needed.

Helpful hints/notes: Advertise and promote this activity during groups, during activity assessments, during resident council meetings and at other meetings, through your therapy department, within your activities schedule of events, and/or in your facility newsletter. Consult a doctor to ensure safety for each participant. Make sure the floor is not slippery. Have participants wear comfortable shoes and clothing. Make sure participants drink plenty of water and take frequent breaks. Invite a martial arts instructor for demonstrations and advice in setting up a safe and effective program for participants.

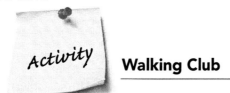

Walking Club

Target audience: Younger residents and short-term stay rehab residents

Objectives/outcomes:

- To build staff and resident rapport

- To help build relationships among residents with similar interests and abilities

- To provide an opportunity for socialization

- To enhance therapy goals

- To promote a healthy lifestyle

- To build strength and endurance and help residents regain their independence

Recommended group size: Independent, in halls

Suggested time frame: Depends on individual abilities of residents

Special needs/ability level (physical/cognitive skills needed): Individuals who can walk independently or with an assistive device (walker, cane) independently. Individuals who have the cognitive capacity to follow a predetermined route.

Activity outline:

- Establish and mark a walking club route. You may mark the route with interesting signs, shapes of shoes, or whatever system works for your facility and residents.

- Have the therapy department assist you in measuring distances so that residents can track their distance.

- Use a form for residents to track their individual progress.

- Encourage residents to "buddy up" with a peer(s) for socialization and support.

- Offer a monthly, daily, or weekly contest of who puts in the most "miles" or whatever measuring you decide to use. Give out a healthy prize (granola bars, fruit, etc.) and post the winner's name in a prominent place. (This gives recognition and incentive to all participants to try to win the next time.)

Variations/adaptations/modifications: Residents who need stand by assistance of one could be assisted to participate with a staff member or assigned volunteer, or even a family member. You will need to know the individual abilities of each resident and make the needed modifications.

Helpful hints/notes: Advertise and promote this activity during groups, during activity assessments, during resident council meetings and at other meetings, through your therapy department, within your activities schedule of events, and/or in your facility newsletter. Consult a doctor to ensure safety for all participants. Make sure the floor is not slippery and the route is safe and free from obstacles. Have participants wear comfortable shoes and clothing. Make sure participants drink plenty of water and take frequent breaks.

Weekend Trivia

Target audience: Younger residents and short-term stay rehab residents

Objectives/outcomes:

- To provide and promote meaningful leisure pursuits

- To stimulate mental functioning

- To promote independence in structuring day

Recommended group size: Independent, in-room

Suggested time frame: Not applicable

Special needs/ability level (physical/cognitive skills needed): Ability to read and write, cognitive skills, thinking skills, ability to pursue leisure interests independently

Activity outline:

- Find a resource for crosswords, word searches, or trivia. Resources include books (you can find them at Wal-Mart and at dollar discount stores) and the Internet. One Internet site to use is *www.dellmagazines.com/*.

- Make a packet of two to three (minimum) puzzles.

- Run off a predetermined number of copies (enough to accommodate the number of residents who want to take part; you will come to know this through your resident assessments).

- Deliver the packets to each resident (as a mail delivery) on Friday afternoons. Turn this into a social visit as well.

- Post the answer page(s) the following Monday in a predetermined areas(s).

- Provide this activity on Friday, to be completed over the weekend.

Variations/adaptations/modifications: Residents who are blind or have limited vision can have staff members, volunteers, or family members read the questions to them and they can provide the answers. You can also pair up roommates/peers to assist one another. Residents can work on the questions as a group while in therapy together or when they are sitting together at meal time. Residents who like to use the computer can go online and get their own puzzles. You can also display a daily trivia board (in a high-traffic area where residents can see it daily). On it, you can post a daily trivia question, and then post the answer and a new question the following day. You can turn this into a contest and have residents submit their written answers in a box, and then draw a name from the winning entries. Open the contest to residents, family members, volunteers, and staff members. This activity promotes daily discussion among staff members, family members, volunteers and residents. You may be surprised at how popular this activity can be.

Helpful hints/notes: Advertise and promote this activity during groups, during activity assessments, during resident council meetings and at other meetings, within your activities schedule of events, and/or in your facility newsletter. Remember to observe all copyright laws.

Welcome Initiative

Target audience: Younger residents and short-term stay rehab residents

Objectives/outcomes:

- To provide a warm welcome to new residents

- To provide comfort and adjustment for new residents

- To ensure that new residents' needs are being met

- To address any concerns or issues immediately

- To provide important information about the facility

- To build staff and resident rapport

Recommended group size: Independent, in-room

Suggested time frame: Length should be based on need and situation. Visits should occur three times during the first week, two times during the second week, and weekly throughout the duration of the resident's stay.

Special needs/ability level (physical/cognitive skills needed): Individuals of all levels should be included.

Activity outline:

- Set this up to be a facility department head/department manager's activity.

- Assign all new residents to a department head on a rotating basis.

- The assigned department head brings a "welcome" plant and Beanie Baby to the new resident and visits with him or her within the first day or two. (Providing the plant/ stuffed animal is optional.)

- The department head should introduce him or herself, and warmly greet and welcome the resident. Ask how things are going and ask pointed questions related to care, food, sleep, therapies, activities, individual needs, any concerns the resident may have, and so on.

- The department head should either address any concerns or issues if able, or take them to the appropriate department for a solution. On the next visit, he or she should inform the resident of the solution or progress made.

- During each visit, revisit the same topics and additional topics as brought forth by discussion.

- Provide this activity to all new admissions.

Variations/adaptations/modifications: You could extend this to include other key staff members.

Helpful hints/notes: Staff interpersonal skills need to be considered when selecting staff members to be included in the delivery of this service. The staff needs to be fully aware of the purpose of this activity and must support its goals. A positive outlook and frame of mind are necessary, as is the ability to seek solutions, address concerns, and maintain a respectful relationship.

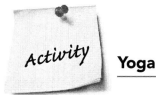

Yoga

Target audience: Younger residents and short-term stay rehab residents

Objectives/outcomes:

- To build staff and resident rapport

- To help build relationships among residents with similar interests and abilities

- To provide an opportunity for socialization

- To enhance therapy goals

- To promote a healthy lifestyle

- To improve balance and reduce the risk of falls

- To improve mobility, flexibility, and function

- To improve coordination

- To improve mind-body coordination

- To decrease joint pain

- To promote relaxation

- To alleviate chronic pain

- To improve sleep

- To reduce stiffness

- To help prevent bone loss

- To improve blood pressure and circulation

- To decrease depression

- To improve cognition and short-term memory

- To enhance vitality and energy

- To improve quality of life on all levels: physical, emotional, mental, and spiritual

- To build strength and endurance and help residents regain their independence

Recommended group size: Can vary, but should be manageable to the leader

Suggested time frame: 30 – 45 minutes

Special needs/ability level (physical/cognitive skills needed): Individuals who can follow actions and physically complete a series of movements

Activity outline:

- Yoga involves slow, conscious breathing, poses, and postures that are safe for all to perform at any age. Yoga will relax the body, ease the mind, and refresh the spirit. Play some relaxing classical music in the background. Read the following steps aloud and demonstrate actions for participants to follow.

- Begin with yoga breathing. Yoga breathing is breathing more deeply than your usual involuntary breathing. By beginning with a breathing sequence, you are increasing your mind's capacity to focus attention on the postures. As you follow the postures, continue to focus on your breathing. While sitting up straight in a chair, put your hands in the prayer position in front of your chest. Relax your feet flat on the floor. Close your eyes and take a deep breath in and slowly exhale. Repeat this five times. As you breathe in and out through your nose, focus on your breath and notice how you are feeling. Become aware of any tension and, as you breathe out, imagine the tension flowing out with the breath. As you breathe in, feel yourself filling up with positive, healing energy. Next, place your hands on your abdomen, one over the other and with palms down, and exhale slowly and completely. Then inhale, breathing into your abdomen. Allow your abdomen to rise and fill like a balloon. Hold your breath in momentarily, and then slowly exhale. Breathe into the abdomen up to five times.

- Limbering (gentle exercises): While sitting in a chair with your feet relaxed on the floor, put your arms down at your sides. Slowly exhale. Inhale as you slowly stretch your arms over your head, lengthening your whole body and stretching from your fingertips to your toes. Exhale as you lift your arms up to the ceiling and down to your sides again. Repeat five times. Inhale as you draw your right knee toward your chest and place your hands around your knee. Exhale as you bend your head toward your knee, tucking your chin into your chest, and hold for a moment. Then release your knee and raise your head from your chest. Repeat with the left knee. Repeat the entire sequence once more.

- Stretches and poses: Place your hands on your thighs just above your knees, with your knees together. Inhale and stretch your arms up and forward and continue the stretch until your arms are above your head. Exhale as you bring your arms back down into the starting position. Repeat five times.

- Sit with your feet relaxed on the floor and your hands on your thighs. Inhale as you slowly bend forward, sliding your hands down your legs to your ankles. Exhale as you slowly return to a sitting position. Repeat five times.

- Sit with your feet relaxed on the floor and your hands hanging down at your sides. Inhale as you slowly relax your body forward. Rest and hold this position for five breaths and return to a sitting position. Repeat once more.

- Sit with your feet relaxed on the floor. Cross your arms in front of your chest. Inhale as you bend forward, touching your elbows to your knees. Exhale as you rise to a sitting position. Repeat five times. On the last sequence, let your arms fall to the floor (hands down), totally relax your body, and breathe in and out for five breaths. Slowly return to a sitting position on the last inhale.

- Shoulder rotations: Sit up straight in a chair, with your arms hanging relaxed at your sides and your feet flat on the floor. Inhale as you bring your shoulders up and to your ears. Roll your shoulders back firmly. Squeeze them as close together as you can. Then exhale as you roll them downward and return to the starting position. Inhale as you squeeze your shoulders together behind you. Bring them up to your ears, and exhale as you roll them forward and down. Continue rotating your shoulders up to five times forward and five times backward.

- Sit with your feet relaxed on the floor and your arms relaxed by your sides. Look straight ahead and gently lift your left knee as high as you can. Hold for up to five breaths. Repeat with your right knee.

- Sit with your feet relaxed on the floor and your arms down at your sides. As you inhale, lift your arms above your head with your hands in a prayer position. Hold for up to five breaths. On each breath, slowly bring your arms down in front of your chest in a prayer position.

- Sit with your feet relaxed on the floor and your arms straight out at your sides, palms down. Inhale as you rotate your palms up and your shoulders roll back. Exhale and roll your palms back down. Repeat five times. Put both arms back out at your sides. Inhale as you slowly lean to the right and your right arm goes down and your left arm goes up (think airplane). Exhale as you come back up to the starting position. Repeat on the left side.

- Twisting pose: Sit with your feet relaxed on the floor and your hands on your knees. Inhale and slowly twist your body to left, exhale, and return to the front. Inhale and slowly twist your body to the right, exhale, and return to the front. Repeat five times.

- Hand to foot: Sit with your feet relaxed on the floor and your hands on your knees. Exhale as you raise both legs and reach toward your feet with your hands/arms. Inhale as you return to the starting position. Repeat five times.

- Sitting up straight in a chair, put your hands in a prayer position in front of your chest. Relax your feet flat on the floor. Close your eyes and take a deep breath in and slowly exhale. Repeat this five times.

- Sun salutation: Sitting up straight in a chair with your feet relaxed on the floor and your hands in a prayer position, inhale and bring your arms up over your head. Exhale as you bring your arms down and around and back into a prayer position in front of your chest. Repeat five times.

- Meditation: Close your eyes, put your hands on your thighs, relax, and focus on your breathing. Bring your attention inward, away from the external world. Soften your face; relax your neck and shoulders. Breathe evenly and slowly. Let your thoughts come and go. Your mind is a beautiful, clear blue sky and your thoughts are white clouds passing across it. Allow a sense of peace and well-being to expand as your mind clears and becomes quiet. Slowly open your eyes.

Variations/adaptations/modifications: Residents who sit in wheelchairs can perform breathing, adapted poses, and postures from a sitting position with a leader's help. You will need to know the individual abilities of each resident and provide the needed modifications.

Provide verbal and visual cues. Simplify movements as needed. Individuals vary in strength and flexibility, so the practice of yoga will be unique to each individual. Allow participants to proceed at their own pace.

Helpful hints/notes: Advertise and promote this activity during groups, during activity assessments, during resident council meetings and at other meetings, through your therapy department, within your activities schedule of events, and/or in your facility newsletter. Consult a doctor to ensure safety for each participant. Have participants wear comfortable clothing. Make sure participants drink plenty of water and take frequent breaks.

Chapter 7

Activities for Men

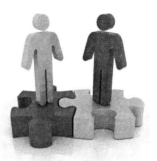

Providing activities that are appealing to men can present a special kind of challenge for activities professionals. This is typically due to two reasons. One, many traditional nursing home activities are naturally centered on activities that appeal to women. Two, men tend to be harder to motivate to take part in large group activities, as they tend not to be as social as women.

The challenges, then, are to develop programs that naturally appeal to men and to find a way to motivate them to participate in these programs. A good place to start is individual assessments to identify the leisure interests of the men in your facility; you can then develop programs from there.

One of the easiest ways to promote more male-oriented events is to establish a Men's Club or a Romeo Club to which only men are invited. Many men were once members of civic organizations or clubs (the Moose Lodge, AMVETS, American Legion, Knights of Columbus, card clubs, golf clubs, etc.), and this will promote friendships and allow the men in your facility to carry on a lifelong tradition of getting together with a group of male friends/peers. Make sure they meet regularly and that a part of each get-together includes discussing what they would like to do the next time they meet. Getting their input ensures their interest and guarantees their participation. Once this formal group is established, they will just naturally gravitate together informally on a regular basis.

The old saying, "The way to a man's heart is through his stomach," holds true not only for new brides but also for activities professionals. Men like to eat! So, any activity that has food as part of the deal is usually well received (e.g., a special men-only dinner out, a monthly men-only breakfast (have the administrator and Activities Department plan and cook the meal in their presence), a monthly men only eat-in (order food from Subway, a pizza place, Kentucky Fried Chicken, etc.), and a men only barbeque on the patio. Men also tend to be competitive, so any activity that allows them to be competitive is usually well received. These can include recreational games (e.g., bowling, basketball, horseshoes, darts, disc golf, or golf putting), trivia contests or other contests, and Wii games or other video games. Special trips/outings that are geared to their former lifestyle are also well received (e.g., taking trips to the "Men's Mall" – Menards, Fleet Farm or the like, visiting a car/truck dealership, driving by the "old farmstead," visiting a working farm, going on fishing trips, and picnicking in the park). Many men also take great pride in their past occupations and in being in the service, so having men gather in a small group to discuss these interests can bring a source of pride to their day. Encourage men to gather together informally to watch whatever sports are of interest on the big screen in the activity area (if you have one). Serve refreshments (beer anyone?) and check in with them periodically to see how the game/race is going. This does not require that a staff person be present continuously. Have men from the community come in and demonstrate or display items and talk with your male residents (e.g., a woodcarver, woodworker, train collector, coin collector, stamp collector, etc.).

In the past, men would gather at the barbershop, corner store, or a coffee shop to "shoot the breeze." So, develop areas where men can gather informally on their own to talk, just like the good old days (e.g., a corner in the main dining room or activity area, the patio in warmer weather, or by the front entrance, either indoors or outdoors, so that they can greet and gab with visitors as they come and go, kind of like sitting outside the old barbershop watching the world go by).

Men also like to help others and to take charge. Create opportunities for them to be of service, and let them host an activity such as an ice cream social or cocktail party. Have them plant a tree for Arbor Day, let them help take care of garden areas throughout the gardening season, and if there is construction going on or the lawn is being mowed, let them gather and watch what's happening. Turn it into an opportunity for an informal activity and bring out the iced tea and lemonade. Spontaneity often breeds the most successful and enjoyable activities.

With a little forethought and imagination you can plan activities that men will enjoy and look forward to. Use the following activities as part of your programming for men.

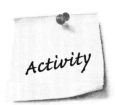

Activity | **6, 5, 4 Dice Game**

Target audience: Men's Club activity

Objectives/outcomes:

- Promotes social interaction between male peers and the staff

- Provides for development of friendships, companionship, and conversation

- Promotes reminiscence, mental stimulation, long-term memory skills, and cognitive/ thinking skills

- Provides a learning opportunity

- Provides an opportunity for recognition

- Maintains and improves fine motor skills

- Maintains and improves hand-eye coordination

- Develops a sense of pride and self-esteem associated with friendly competition and team play

Recommended group size: Small to medium (no more than 10 – 15)

Suggested time frame: One hour

Special needs/ability level (physical/cognitive skills needed): Primarily residents with moderate to high cognitive functioning. Ability to follow directions, complete tasks, respond verbally, and interact on some level.

Activity outline:

- You will need five dice and a cup to hold them.

- Arrange participants around table(s).

- Explain the object of the game. All participants will have a turn rolling the dice for up to three rolls (depending on what they roll). The object is to shake a 6, 5, and 4 in successive order. You must roll a 6 on the first roll to get another roll. Then you must roll a 5 to get your third and final roll. You must get a 4 on this roll (so that you have a 6, 5, 4) by the third roll to be in the game. Add the total of the other two dice to get your score. Go around to each participant; the person with the highest score (of those getting a score) is the winner of that round. Play as many rounds as you can in 45 minutes, given the number of participants (reserve 15 minutes for refreshments at the end). Here are some examples to further explain how the game is played:

- A 6 and a 5 are rolled on the first round. The 6 and 5 are saved and the remaining three dice are rolled again. A 4 and two other numbers are rolled. The 4 is saved and the remaining two dice are rolled again (or the other two numbers can be saved if they equal a high score, in which case the third roll is not required). On the third roll, a 6 and a 4 are rolled. The score is 10 for this participant.

- On the first roll, no 6 is rolled. This ends this participant's turn; to stay in the game you must roll a 6, 5, and 4 successively.

- A 6, 5, and 4 are all rolled on the first roll. The player would save all of these and has the option of rolling the other two dice again to get a higher score. (Note that you cannot save a 5 and a 4 if a 6 is not rolled; they have to be rolled in succession.) If this player rolls two more times in an attempt to get a higher score and ends up rolling a 6 and a 1 on the second roll (for a score of 7), he can save both or roll again. He cannot save just the 6 (because this is the highest you can roll) and roll one die. He must save both or roll both again.

• Be sure to praise all efforts and participation throughout the game, not just success, and again at the end of the game.

• Thank everyone for participating and for his good sportsmanship.

• Serve refreshments at the end (this eliminates the possibility of spills and dirty dice while playing). Offer items such as soda, beer, chips, pretzels, peanuts, and popcorn.

Variations/adaptations/modifications: You will need to offer more assistance to residents with diminished abilities (they may be able to roll dice but not add or comprehend when play ends; you can give gentle reminders along with additional verbal and visual cues). This activity can include low-functioning residents when adaptations/modifications are made.

Helpful hints/notes: Much of the setup for this event can be done prior to gathering residents so that you are ready to begin once residents have gathered. Assemble all needed equipment and supplies prior to the start of the activity. Encourage a positive atmosphere for fair, fun recreational play and competition. Observe all infection-control guidelines and individual resident dietary needs/restrictions when serving food and beverages.

Men's Card Club

Target audience: Men's Club activity

Objectives/outcomes:

- Promotes social interaction between male peers and the staff

- Provides for development of friendships, companionship, and conversation

- Promotes reminiscence, mental stimulation, long-term memory skills, and cognitive/thinking skills

- Provides a learning opportunity

- Provides an opportunity for recognition

- Maintains and improves fine motor skills

- Maintains and improves hand-eye coordination

- Develops a sense of pride and self-esteem associated with friendly competition and team play

Recommended group size: Small to medium

Suggested time frame: One hour

Special needs/ability level (physical/cognitive skills needed): Primarily residents with moderate to high cognitive functioning. Must know card games or be able to learn card games. Ability to follow directions, complete tasks, respond verbally, and interact on some level.

Activity outline:

- You will need decks of cards and paper and pens for keeping score as needed.

- Arrange participants around table(s) according to the number of players for each card game (as some card games require a certain number of players), and according to what card game each participant knows how to play or wants to learn. Pair up new learners with the "experts" on each card game.

- The participants' interests dictate the types of card games played. Some popular card games include Uno, sheep's head, smear, canasta, kings korners, crazy eights, hearts, poker, cribbage (you will need a cribbage board), war, 500 rummy, pinochle (you will need a pinochle deck), spoons, black jack, and dirty clubs.

- Be sure to praise all efforts and participation throughout the game, not just success, and again at the end of the game.

- Thank everyone for participating and for his good sportsmanship.

- Serve refreshments at the end (this eliminates the possibility of spills and dirty cards while playing). Offer items such as soda, beer, chips, pretzels, peanuts, and popcorn.

Variations/adaptations/modifications: You will need to offer more assistance to residents with diminished abilities (they may be able to play with staff assistance; gentle reminders can be given along with additional verbal and visual cues). Some participants may need adaptive equipment in the form of cardholders.

Helpful hints/notes: Much of the setup for this event can be done prior to gathering residents so that you are ready to begin once residents have gathered. Assemble all needed equipment and supplies prior to the start of the activity. Encourage a positive atmosphere for fair, fun recreational play and competition. Observe all infection-control guidelines and individual resident dietary needs/restrictions when serving food and beverages.

Men's Club Breakfast/Luncheon

Target audience: Men's Club activity

Objectives/outcomes:

- Promotes social interaction between male peers and the staff

- Promotes camaraderie, a good time, sharing of stories, and good food

- Provides an opportunity to shoot the breeze with the guys

- Provides for development of friendships, companionship, and conversation

- Provides an opportunity to meet other men with similar or varying interests

- Promotes reminiscence

Recommended group size: Small to medium

Suggested time frame: One hour, or as needed

Special needs/ability level (physical/cognitive skills needed): Primarily residents with moderate to high cognitive functioning

Activity outline:

- Schedule a special breakfast or luncheon just for men. You will need to provide a list of participants to the dietary and nursing staffs.

- For a breakfast, plan and coordinate the menu with the Dietary Department. Get needed supplies from that department. A baked egg dish, hash browns in the oven, bacon done in the oven, and pancakes done on the griddle are all great breakfast options for men. Men tend to like hearty breakfasts.

- Make all or part of the meal with the participants already gathered together (if they are able, they can prepare some of it). This way, they get to enjoy the aroma and can be served while the food is hot. Make sure to give them coffee and juice while they wait for the food to be prepared.

- Promote conversation throughout the get-together.

- Invite the administrator to share a leisurely breakfast with the men.

- For a luncheon, order in food, let the men pick each time the restaurant from which they would like to order the food, and vary it from time to time. Sub sandwiches, burgers and fries, fish, chicken dinners, Chinese food, and pizza are usually well-received menu options. Get copies of menus from the places you routinely order from so that residents can make their own selections. If it's an option, have the food delivered; otherwise, you will need to assign a staff member to pick up the food.

- Invite the administrator to share the luncheon with the men.

Variations/adaptations/modifications: For a luncheon, you could also select a menu and have the men prepare and eat it together (e.g., a chili luncheon). Secure needed supplies from the Dietary Department.

Helpful hints/notes: Much of the setup for this event can be done prior to gathering residents so that you are ready to begin once residents have gathered. Assemble all needed equipment and supplies prior to the start of the activity. Observe all infection-control guidelines and individual resident dietary needs/restrictions when serving food and beverages.

Men's Club Grill-Out or Picnic

Target audience: Men's Club activity

Objectives/outcomes:

- Promotes social interaction between male peers and the staff

- Promotes camaraderie, a good time, sharing of stories, and good food

- Provides an opportunity to shoot the breeze with the guys

- Provides for development of friendships, companionship, and conversation

- Provides an opportunity to meet other men with similar or varying interests

- Promotes reminiscence

Recommended group size: Small to medium

Suggested time frame: One hour, or as needed

Special needs/ability level (physical/cognitive skills needed): Primarily residents with moderate to high cognitive functioning

Activity outline:

- Schedule a grill-out on the patio or a picnic just for the men. You will need to provide a list of participants to the dietary and nursing staffs. Schedule any needed volunteer helpers.

- For a grill-out, have the men plan the menu and coordinate needed supplies through the Dietary Department. Some good options are hamburgers, bratwurst, buns, potato salad, baked beans, chips, cookies or bars, and lemonade.

- Gather the men together to sit and converse (provide the lemonade) while the meat is being grilled. (Have the dietary staff supply the rest of the items already made.)

- Promote conversation throughout the get-together.

- For a picnic in the park, order the food, let the men choose from which restaurant they would like to order, and vary it from time to time. Pick up the food on your way to the park. Sub sandwiches, burgers and fries, and chicken dinners are usually well-received menu options for picnics. Get copies of menus from the places you routinely order from so that residents can make their own selections. The men may enjoy having beer on a picnic as well as soda. Let the men pick what handicapped-accessible park to visit each time. Don't forget bug spray, sunscreen, disposable dishware, serving utensils, grilling supplies, wet wipes, and any other items you may need for a picnic. Make and keep a master list for outings to use each time.

Variations/adaptations/modifications: For a picnic, you could also have the men prepare sub sandwiches or you could take the food to grill once you are at the park. Secure needed supplies from the Dietary Department.

Helpful hints/notes: Much of the setup for this activity can be done prior to gathering residents so that you are ready to begin once residents have gathered. Assemble all needed equipment and supplies prior to the start of the activity. Observe all infection-control guidelines and individual resident dietary needs/restrictions when serving food and beverages. Also, plan ahead to ensure the picnic tables are available.

Men's Gathering/Coffee and Gab Session

Target audience: Men's Club activity

Objectives/outcomes:

- Promotes social interaction between male peers and the staff

- Provides an opportunity to shoot the breeze in a less structured environment, and for participants to determine the flow of the session

- Provides for development of friendships, companionship, and conversation

- Promotes reminiscence, mental stimulation, long-term memory skills, and cognitive/ thinking skills

- Provides a learning opportunity

Recommended group size: Small to medium

Suggested time frame: 30 minutes

Special needs/ability level (physical/cognitive skills needed): Primarily residents with moderate to high cognitive functioning. Ability to reminisce, respond verbally, and interact on some level.

Activity outline:

- Hold this session early to mid-morning; it's more of a wakeup activity just for men to get together informally on a routine basis (it could be daily, weekly, or monthly). Once it is held for awhile with staff assistance, you may find that it can take on a life of its own and the men will gather on their own and not need the staff to assist beyond maybe providing them the coffee and refreshments and just stopping by or checking in on them from time to time.

- Serve coffee and refreshments (vary what you serve)—for example, muffins, coffee cake, donuts, rolls, bagels, cookies, and so on.

- Allow them to discuss whatever comes up. You may need to initially get the conversation going by discussing upcoming events, holidays, weather, and so on. But allow the conversation to go in whatever direction the men take it; remember that this is an informal activity.

- Allow the gathering to just naturally come to an end as you direct them to other planned activities or independent leisure pursuits for the day.

Variations/adaptations/modifications: You may want to assign a male volunteer, male resident, or staff member to oversee this gathering. For variation, you may want to start the gathering with a preplanned topic of discussion; for example, you could use the newspaper to come up with a topic. This activity works well in conjunction with a continental breakfast, which more facilities are going to, so if your facility offers this turn it into an activity as well by grouping male peers together.

Helpful hints/notes: Much of the setup for this activity can be done prior to gathering residents so that you are ready to begin once residents have gathered. Assemble all needed equipment and supplies prior to the start of the activity. Observe all infection-control guidelines and individual resident dietary needs/restrictions when serving food and beverages.

Romeo Club

Target audience: Men's Club activity

Objectives/outcomes:

- Promotes social interaction between male peers and the staff

- Promotes camaraderie, a good time, sharing of stories, and (often) good food

- Provides an opportunity to shoot the breeze with the guys

- Provides for development of friendships, companionship, and conversation

- Provides an opportunity to meet other men with similar or varying interests

- Promotes reminiscence, mental stimulation, long-term memory skills, and cognitive/thinking skills

- Provides a learning opportunity

- Provides an opportunity for recognition and to feel special (after all, what man doesn't want to be a Romeo?)

Recommended group size: Small to medium

Suggested time frame: One hour

Special needs/ability level (physical/cognitive skills needed): Primarily residents with moderate to high cognitive functioning. Ability to reminisce, respond verbally, interact on some level, and complete tasks.

Activity outline:

- Hold the Romeo Club at least monthly. Have the Romeo members decide what they will do each month.

- Here's a little history of Romeo Clubs. Tom Brokaw gave the name "Romeo" notoriety in his book *The Greatest Generation*. There are several stories regarding how the

Romeos originated. One such story says that John "Lefty" Caulfield (a school principal and U.S. Navy retiree) started the first Romeo Club at various diners in Cambridge, Mass., and dubbed it "Retired Old Men Eating Out." The clubs give men an opportunity to meet with other men and enjoy good food and conversation.

- You will need to establish your Romeo Club members and an acronym that fits your group. You may not want it to be "Retired Old Men Eating Out," as you will most likely take part in other events besides dining out. One option would be "Retired Older Men Enjoying Opportunities. "Older" sounds more positive than "old" and "enjoying opportunities" describes the purpose of the group.

- Have each member wear a red baseball cap with the word *ROMEO* embroidered on it. Or have the Romeos themselves write the word *ROMEO* on their own hat with fabric paint. This could be your initial activity when you get the group going.

- Have the Romeos plan out their monthly activities; you may need to give them some ideas initially to get them started. Some successful ideas include dining out, special luncheons or breakfasts, bus rides or trips, recreational games, card games, picnics, cookouts, going to ballgames, hosting activities for other residents, meeting jointly with the women's Red Hat Club a couple of times per year for socials, inviting community Romeo groups to visit the facility for a joint activity, and virtually any activity that a Men's Club would enjoy.

Variations/adaptations/modifications: You may want to assign a male volunteer, male resident, or staff member (how about a male administrator?) to oversee the club.

Helpful hints/notes: Much of the setup for this activity can be done prior to gathering residents so that you are ready to begin once residents have gathered. Assemble all needed equipment and supplies prior to the start of the activity. Observe all infection-control guidelines and individual resident dietary needs/restrictions when serving food and beverages.

Turkey Shoot

Target audience: Men's Club activity

Objectives/outcomes:

- Promotes social interaction between male peers and the staff

- Provides for development of friendships, companionship, and conversation

- Promotes reminiscence, mental stimulation, long-term memory skills, and cognitive/thinking skills

- Provides a learning opportunity

- Provides an opportunity for recognition

- Provide opportunities for physical exercise and friendly competition in a recreational setting

- Maintains and improves fine and gross motor skills

- Maintains and improves hand-eye coordination

- Develops a sense of pride and self-esteem associated with friendly competition and team play

Recommended group size: Small to large

Suggested time frame: One hour

Special needs/ability level (physical/cognitive skills needed): Primarily residents with moderate to high cognitive functioning. Ability to follow directions, complete tasks, respond verbally, and interact on some level.

Activity outline:

- You will need "turkeys" (turkey shapes cut out of construction paper) that have numbers on them for scoring points (5, 10, 15, 20, 25), a dart board (or a cork board or some board that turkeys can be stapled to and that darts can be thrown at and stick to), and darts. (Set up the board prior to the start of the activity.)

- Each participant should be given a predetermined number of darts (e.g., five). The object of the game is for them to throw the darts at the board, aiming for the turkeys. Once they have thrown their darts, add up the scores and keep a running tally for each round. Complete as many rounds as you can, based on the number of participants and the amount of time allotted for the activity. The participant with the highest score of the total of all rounds at the end of the game is the winner.

- Announce first, second, and third place winners. Let every participant know his score at the end of the game.

- Be sure to praise all efforts and participation throughout the game, not just success, and again at the end of the game.

- Thank everyone for participating and for his good sportsmanship.

Variations/adaptations/modifications: You will need to simplify tasks, make adaptations (they may need closer targets, or verbal and visual cues), and offer more assistance to residents with diminished abilities (they may be able to perform tasks with direct hand-over-hand guidance). Some residents may need to sit closer to the target, but do not make it too easy, as you want there to be some challenge and yet some success. This activity can include low-functioning residents when adaptations/modifications are made. As a variation, change the targets on the board (to rabbits, fish, deer, etc.) to coordinate with the season and what may be "hunted" or "caught" at any particular time.

Helpful hints/notes: Much of the setup for this event can be done prior to gathering residents so that you are ready to begin once residents have gathered. Assemble all needed equipment and supplies prior to the start of the activity. Encourage a positive atmosphere for fair, fun recreational play and competition. Observe safety with the use of darts by setting up the target in an area where no one will be walking behind it. Keep all participants a safe distance away from flying darts and provide supervision throughout to maintain safety.

Chapter 8

Activities for Women

Providing activities that appeal to women is usually pretty easy. This is because many traditional nursing home activities are naturally centered on activities that appeal to women, and because women tend to be very social by nature.

Some activities, however, are geared specifically to women, and most men would not care to participate in them or appreciate them as much as women do. Some of these activities include joining a Red Hat Society, tea socials, fondue parties, gourmet coffee socials, shopping trips, spa days, Pampered Chef demonstrations, home decorating demonstrations, Mary Kay facials, quilting demonstrations, cooking clubs, fashion shows, manicures, scrapbooking, and crafts.

Be sure to look at the individual assessments of the women in your facility to determine what they enjoy as leisure activities; then you can develop programs from there. Women are traditionally caretakers and nurturers. Therefore, women tend to enjoy activities that allow them to care for or nurture something, including the following:

- Gardening

- Caring for house plants

- Volunteer roles such as calling bingo

- Assisting with facility mailings

- Helping to serve or clean up after social activities

- Preparing snacks

- Creating scrapbooks containing pictures of residents involved in activities at the facility

- Leading discussion or reading groups

- Taking apart donated funeral bouquets and arranging them in vases for the dining room tables

- Helping with church services or conducting a rosary or devotional in a small group

Encouraging women residents to take on leadership roles, including leading or assisting with group activities, is one way to build their self-esteem (this is true for men as well). Remember that activities do not have to be conducted by the activities staff. Utilize residents who have held leadership roles within the community, and allow them to continue to enjoy leadership roles in their "new community" by providing activities to their peers. Because women are more social than men, they usually enjoy any activities that are social in nature. And women, just like men, enjoy food! Hence, offer picnics, grill-outs, dining excursions, and special luncheons/eat-ins just for them.

One of the easiest ways to promote more female-oriented events is to establish a Women's Club, or better yet, a Red Hat Society to which only women are invited. Many women previously were members of civic organizations or clubs (the Moose Lodge, American Legion, card clubs, golf clubs, homemakers' clubs, church groups, sewing circles, quilting and craft clubs, etc.), and this will promote friendships and allow women to carry on a lifelong tradition of getting together with a group of female friends/peers. Make sure they meet regularly and that a part of each get-together includes discussing what they would like to do the next time they meet. Getting their input ensures their interest and guarantees their participation. Once this formal group is established, they will just naturally gravitate together informally on a regular basis.

With a little forethought and imagination you can plan activities that women will enjoy and look forward to. Use the following activities as part of your programming for women.

Activity | **Cooking Club**

Target audience: Women who enjoy cooking (some men might enjoy this as well)

Objectives/outcomes:

- Promotes social interaction between peers and the staff

- Provides for development of friendships, companionship, and conversation

- Promotes reminiscence, mental stimulation, long-term memory skills, and cognitive/thinking skills

- Promotes creative expression and choice

- Provides a learning opportunity

Recommended group size: Small to medium (maximum of 12 – 15)

Suggested time frame: One hour, or as needed

Special needs/ability level (physical/cognitive skills needed): Primarily residents with moderate to high cognitive functioning

Activity outline:

- Hold this activity weekly or on a routine basis as dictated by participant interest.

- Have participants look through recipe books or bring their favorite recipes to choose from. Try all sorts of recipes (e.g., soups, salads, stir fry, casseroles, wraps, dips, snacks, muffins, quick breads, cookies, pies, desserts, etc.). You can do this at the conclusion of each session so that you have the recipe selected for the next session. One caveat: You must be able to complete and serve the recipe in the time allotted for this activity. Or you can make the recipe in the morning and serve the food at an afternoon activity.

- Either shop for or secure the needed items from the Dietary Department.

- Have all residents wash their hands prior to preparing food.

- Follow and prepare the recipe, dividing the tasks among residents (cleaning, chopping, cutting, measuring, stirring, etc.) so that they all have tasks they are capable of completing.

- Reminisce or "gab" while the recipe is cooking or baking.

- Sample the recipe when complete.

- Serve a beverage as well.

- Promote conversation throughout.

Variations/adaptations/modifications: You will need to simplify tasks, make adaptations (built-up utensils, special cutting boards that hold items in place for those who can use only one arm/hand, and additional verbal and visual cues for lower-functioning residents), and give simpler tasks and offer more assistance to residents with diminished abilities, as they may be able to perform tasks with direct hand-over-hand guidance. Some activities can include low-functioning residents when adaptations/modifications are made. It is best to offer two different kinds of cooking activities: a cooking club for more able-bodied participants, and a simple cooking group for low-functioning/dementia participants. If you do not have an activity kitchen you can do "kitchenless" cooking on a cart and take the activity to each unit (you may want to do this on a memory/dementia care unit anyway). You will need to stock your cart with a toaster/convection oven, blender, electric fry pan, utensils, recipe ingredients, and so on. Simpler recipes that can be made with this "portable" setup will need to be selected. There is an advantage to this portable cooking activity: The smells on the unit will draw participants in to sample the recipe, at the very least.

Helpful hints/notes: Make sure participants use caution with sharp knives, and do not leave participants unsupervised. Much of the setup for this activity can be done prior to gathering residents so that you are ready to begin once residents have gathered. Assemble all needed equipment and supplies prior to the start of the activity. Observe all infection-control guidelines and individual resident dietary needs/restrictions when serving food and beverages.

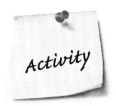

Activity | **Devotional/Prayer Group**

Target audience: Women who are religious and/or who served on church groups

Objectives/outcomes:

- To promote and express faith in an informal setting

- To nurture themselves and others through prayer

- To feel a part of a larger world and a higher power

- To nurture spirituality

- To feel good about themselves and others

Recommended group size: Small, to be more intimate

Suggested time frame: 15 – 30 minutes

Special needs/ability level (physical/cognitive skills needed): All ability levels

Activity outline:

- Hold this on the unit/in a household in a private area to provide a more intimate setting and save on gathering time. You can also utilize the chapel area, but you may spend more time gathering residents and helping them back to their unit than you spend conducting the actual activity.

- Offer this routinely based on resident preference (e.g., daily, weekly, or monthly). Right after breakfast (to get the day started off right) or right before lunch (many residents are just waiting for lunch) are usually good times.

- If possible, secure a volunteer or resident/participant to take this on.

- Have devotional/inspirational books on hand that you can work your way through, sharing a new devotional each time, and adding any personal experiences or antidotes to make it more real.

- Use standard prayers, or if you are comfortable, say your own, and ask participants to say prayers. Be sure to pray for others who are in need.

- Close with the Lord's Prayer.

- Thank participants and inform them of the next devotional.

Helpful hints/notes: Keep devotional/prayer groups nondenominational to encourage participants of all religions to take part.

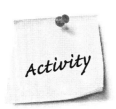

Activity

Fashion Show

Target audience: Women who enjoy fashion

Objectives/outcomes:

- To provide creative and expressive activity for interested residents

- To provide mental stimulation, peer socialization, and recreation

- To provide for companionship and conversation

- To provide an opportunity to reminisce

Recommended group size: Medium to large

Suggested time frame: One hour

Special needs/ability level (physical/cognitive skills needed): None. This is a passive/observing activity for most people.

Activity outline:

- Schedule a fashion show (it's nice to do a spring and a fall fashion show to highlight the new fashions for each season).

- This will require some advanced prep work. Seek staff members, family members, volunteers, and residents who would like to be the models by advertising the event using a poster and sign-up sheet. Have the models select an outfit either from something they have recently purchased or by eliciting a local clothing store to "borrow" outfits for the day. If you choose the latter option, be sure to give the store something in return (e.g., free advertising on your posters, and in your announcements on the day of the event). The models will be responsible either way to get their own outfit(s). In the case of resident models, you will need to schedule a day to visit a local store so that they can select an outfit. Once the models have selected an outfit, they will need to give you a picture or show you the outfit in advance so that whoever is going to be the announcer the day of the event can plan what he or she is going to say about each particular outfit. You will need to also predetermine the order of the models and let them know as well by writing a script and giving copies to all participants so that they can follow along. Because you want the fashion show to last about an hour, plan to have about a dozen outfits modeled. (If you have fewer participants, they can model more than one outfit.)

- The day of the event create a runway by using a roll of flat carpet or a line of mats or something similar to define the area. Play soft background music throughout the program.

- The announcer welcomes everyone to the fashion show and makes any "housekeeping" announcements (e.g., thanking local businesses for allowing the use of their clothing). Then the announcer follows the script; he or she announces the model (as the model walks down the runway and shows off the outfit), describes the outfit, thanks the model, and encourages the audience to applaud in recognition of the model.

- At the conclusion, have all participants come back out and line up. Thank all the participants, the audience, and anyone else who helped with the event, and elicit another round of applause.

- Serve light refreshments to everyone in attendance (e.g., punch and cookies).

- If models "borrowed" outfits from local businesses, they are responsible for returning them to the store. A staff member will need to return any resident outfits for them.

Variations/adaptations/modifications: A variation of this event is to hold a "silly, wacky, or outrageous" fashion show. Adjust the planning accordingly to fit your theme; your goal is strictly to have fun. For this event, participants would need to "create" their outfits (e.g., a spaghetti-strapped dress would have straps made from real strings of spaghetti). Another variation is to hold a period fashion show highlighting fashions from a particular decade in history (e.g., flappers).

Helpful hints/notes: Much of the setup for this event can be done prior to gathering residents so that you are ready to begin once residents have gathered. Assemble all needed equipment and supplies prior to the start of the activity. Observe all infection-control guidelines and individual resident dietary needs/restrictions when serving food and beverages.

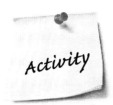

Fondue Party/Social

Target audience: Women's Club activity

Objectives/outcomes:

- Promotes social interaction between female peers and the staff

- Promotes camaraderie, a good time, sharing of stories, and good food

- Provides an opportunity to "gossip" with the "girls"

- Provides for development of friendships, companionship, and conversation

- Provides an opportunity to meet other women with similar or varying interests

- Promotes reminiscence

Recommended group size: Small to medium

Suggested time frame: One hour, or as needed

Special needs/ability level (physical/cognitive skills needed): Primarily residents with moderate to high cognitive functioning

Activity outline:

- Schedule a fondue party/social just for women.

- Fondue is a centuries-old Swiss creation born of a need to make the dried-out winter stores of cheese and bread more palatable. Village peasants would melt the cheese in a communal pot, add wine or brandy, and dip the crusty bread into it. In this way, the first easy fondue recipe was born. The delicious concoction, named *fondue* from the French word meaning to blend or to melt, became both a meal and a social event. Fondue is still a social event, but it is now much more than a peasant's meal. It's a festive dinner, an elegant dessert, and a fun party dip. Even though chocolate fondue recipes were a few hundred years late in getting here, it was worth the wait.

- Select recipes and secure ingredients for the makings of one or several fondues. Either you will need to purchase or secure them through your Dietary Department. You will also need to secure fondue pot(s) or fondue sticks or use toothpicks.

• Make the fondues as part of the activity.

• Let everyone sample the fondues.

• Promote conversation throughout the activity.

• Serve a beverage of choice by the group in attendance (this could be coffee, tea, wine, or punch).

• Play quiet background music to set the mood.

Helpful hints/notes: Ask the staff to borrow fondue pots, pick them up on clearance after the holidays, or look for them at secondhand shops and rummage sales. Much of the setup for the event can be done prior to gathering residents so that you are ready to begin once residents have gathered. Assemble all needed equipment and supplies prior to the start of the activity. Observe all infection-control guidelines and individual resident dietary needs/restrictions when serving food and beverages.

Fondue Recipes:

Classic Cheese Fondue

Traditionally, fondue is made with a blend of Swiss Emmenthal and Gruyère cheeses. Emmenthal is very mild, and Gruyère, especially well-aged Gruyère, is very pungent. A half-and-half mixture is pleasing to most people, but you should feel free to adjust the proportions to your liking.

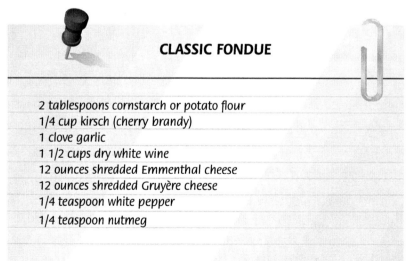

CLASSIC FONDUE

2 tablespoons cornstarch or potato flour
1/4 cup kirsch (cherry brandy)
1 clove garlic
1 1/2 cups dry white wine
12 ounces shredded Emmenthal cheese
12 ounces shredded Gruyère cheese
1/4 teaspoon white pepper
1/4 teaspoon nutmeg

Combine the cornstarch and kirsch. Set aside.

Slice the garlic in half lengthwise and rub the cut side over the inside of a medium-size heavy saucepan. Discard the garlic. Pour the wine into the saucepan and bring it to a boil over a medium-high heat. Immediately reduce the heat to low. Add the cheese to the wine by handfuls and stir slowly until the cheese is just melted. (Stirring in a figure eight or zigzag motion prevents the cheese from clumping.)

Stir in the cornstarch mixture, pepper, and nutmeg. Simmer for two or three minutes until it begins to thicken, but do not let it boil. Transfer to a warmed ceramic fondue pot and serve immediately. Keep warm over a very low flame.

This original/traditional cheese fondue recipe is still best served with the original dipper; serve with two to three loaves of crusty French bread, cut into 1-inch cubes. Serves six.

Variations:
After seasoning the saucepan with garlic, sauté either two cloves of garlic or two shallots, finely chopped in 1 tablespoon of butter and proceed with the recipe.

Tip: Purchase a trial-size bottle of kirsch if you feel the remains of a full bottle will just sit on the shelf.

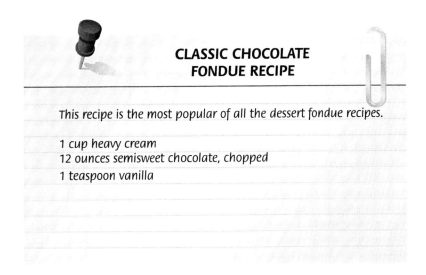

CLASSIC CHOCOLATE FONDUE RECIPE

This recipe is the most popular of all the dessert fondue recipes.

1 cup heavy cream
12 ounces semisweet chocolate, chopped
1 teaspoon vanilla

Heat the cream in a medium saucepan over medium-low heat until hot, about two to three minutes. When hot, add the chocolate and stir until it is just melted and smooth. Stir in vanilla. Transfer to a warm ceramic fondue pot.

Serve with your choice of fresh strawberries, bananas, apple wedges, pound cake, ladyfingers, and almond biscotti. Serves six or more.

Variation:

Substitute 2 to 3 tablespoons of kirsch, brandy, rum, or orange liqueur for the vanilla.

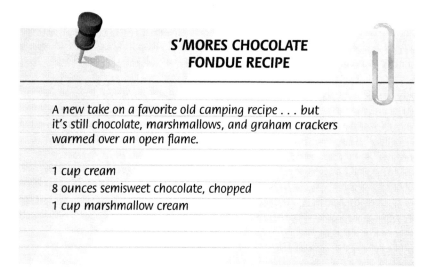

S'MORES CHOCOLATE FONDUE RECIPE

A new take on a favorite old camping recipe . . . but it's still chocolate, marshmallows, and graham crackers warmed over an open flame.

1 cup cream
8 ounces semisweet chocolate, chopped
1 cup marshmallow cream

Slowly warm the cream in a medium saucepan over medium-low heat. When hot, add the chocolate pieces, stirring until melted. Stir in the marshmallow cream and warm the mixture. Transfer to a warm fondue pot.

Serve with graham crackers and marshmallows, of course. Serves six or more.

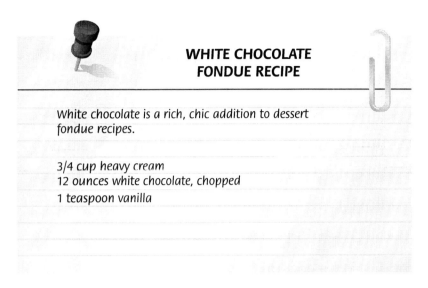

WHITE CHOCOLATE FONDUE RECIPE

White chocolate is a rich, chic addition to dessert fondue recipes.

3/4 cup heavy cream
12 ounces white chocolate, chopped
1 teaspoon vanilla

Heat the cream in a medium saucepan over medium-low heat until hot, about two to three minutes. When hot, add the chocolate and stir until it is just melted and smooth. Stir in vanilla. Transfer to a warm fondue pot.

Serve with your choice of fresh strawberries, bananas, apple wedges, pound cake, ladyfingers, and biscotti. Serves six or more.

Variation:

Substitute 2 to 3 tablespoons of kirsch, brandy, rum, or orange liqueur for the vanilla.

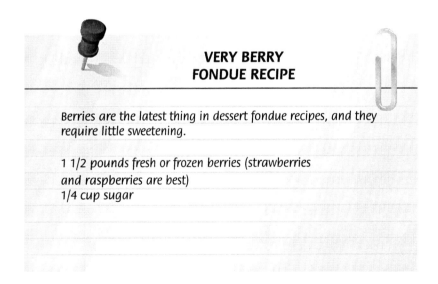

VERY BERRY FONDUE RECIPE

Berries are the latest thing in dessert fondue recipes, and they require little sweetening.

1 1/2 pounds fresh or frozen berries (strawberries and raspberries are best)
1/4 cup sugar

Place the berries in a food processor or blender and puree until smooth. Press the puree through a strainer or cheesecloth (to remove the seeds) and into a medium saucepan. Add the sugar and heat until the sugar has dissolved. Transfer to a warm fondue pot.

This recipe may be prepared two or three days in advance. Serve with shortcake or pound cake, and your choice of cheese cubes. Serves six or more.

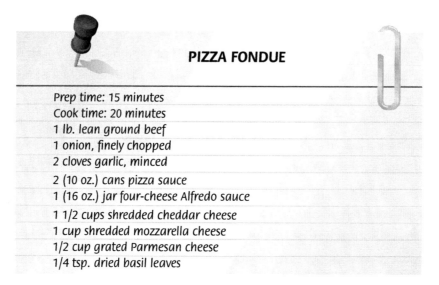

PIZZA FONDUE

Prep time: 15 minutes
Cook time: 20 minutes
1 lb. lean ground beef
1 onion, finely chopped
2 cloves garlic, minced
2 (10 oz.) cans pizza sauce
1 (16 oz.) jar four-cheese Alfredo sauce
1 1/2 cups shredded cheddar cheese
1 cup shredded mozzarella cheese
1/2 cup grated Parmesan cheese
1/4 tsp. dried basil leaves

Brown the ground beef, onion, and garlic in a heavy skillet. Drain well. Add remaining ingredients and cook slowly, stirring frequently, until cheeses melt and mixture is blended. Pour into the fondue pot and serve with breadsticks for dippers, or you can cut pizza dough into wedges, brush with olive oil, and bake until brown and crispy. Serves eight.

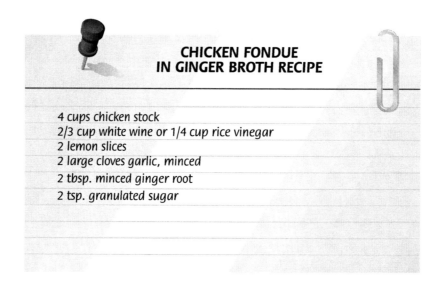

**CHICKEN FONDUE
IN GINGER BROTH RECIPE**

4 cups chicken stock
2/3 cup white wine or 1/4 cup rice vinegar
2 lemon slices
2 large cloves garlic, minced
2 tbsp. minced ginger root
2 tsp. granulated sugar

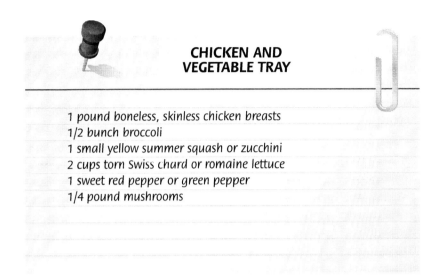

**CHICKEN AND
VEGETABLE TRAY**

1 pound boneless, skinless chicken breasts
1/2 bunch broccoli
1 small yellow summer squash or zucchini
2 cups torn Swiss chard or romaine lettuce
1 sweet red pepper or green pepper
1/4 pound mushrooms

Hot Chili Sauce (recipe follows)

Garlic Sauce (recipe follows)

Fondue Cooking Stock: In a fondue pot, electric skillet, or electric wok, combine chicken stock, white wine, lemon slices, garlic, ginger, and sugar. Just before serving, heat to simmer in fondue pot.

Chicken and Vegetable Tray: Cut chicken into ¾-inch pieces; place on serving platter. Cut broccoli, summer squash, Swiss chard, and sweet pepper into bite-size pieces; arrange along with mushrooms on a separate platter. Using long fondue forks, spear chicken or vegetables; dip into simmering fondue broth to cook. Cook chicken pieces until no longer pink inside and vegetables until tender-crisp. Serve with Hot Chili Sauce and Garlic Sauce for dipping.

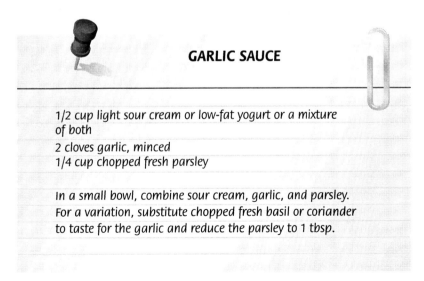

GARLIC SAUCE

1/2 cup light sour cream or low-fat yogurt or a mixture
of both
2 cloves garlic, minced
1/4 cup chopped fresh parsley

In a small bowl, combine sour cream, garlic, and parsley.
For a variation, substitute chopped fresh basil or coriander
to taste for the garlic and reduce the parsley to 1 tbsp.

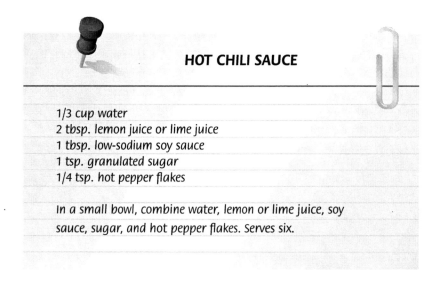

HOT CHILI SAUCE

1/3 cup water
2 tbsp. lemon juice or lime juice
1 tbsp. low-sodium soy sauce
1 tsp. granulated sugar
1/4 tsp. hot pepper flakes

In a small bowl, combine water, lemon or lime juice, soy sauce, sugar, and hot pepper flakes. Serves six.

HOT CRAB FONDUE RECIPE

1 tbsp. unsalted butter
2 tbsp. shallot, minced
3 tbsp. dry white wine
1 cup half-and-half or cream
8 ounces cream cheese, cut into pieces, at room temperature
4 ounces white cheddar cheese, shredded
1/2 pound crab meat

Juice of one lemon	2 tsp. Dijon mustard
1 tsp. Worcestershire sauce	1/2 tsp. Old Bay seasoning

2 cups broccoli florets, blanched and cooled
Breadsticks

In a pot over medium heat, sweat shallots briefly in butter. Add wine, half-and-half, cream cheese, and cheddar cheese. Stir until cheese is melted and mixture is smooth. Stir in remaining ingredients and serve while hot and bubbly with broccoli and breadsticks. Serves two.

SHRIMP FONDUE

1 (10.75 oz.) can condensed cream of shrimp soup
1 (10.75 oz.) can condensed cream of mushroom soup
1 (6 oz.) can tiny shrimp, drained
1 (1 lb.) loaf processed cheese food, cubed
2 packages cocktail rye

In a large saucepan, combine the cream of shrimp soup, cream of mushroom soup, canned shrimp, and cheese. Cook over medium-low heat, stirring frequently, until cheese is melted and well blended. Serve on cocktail rye slices.

Gardening Club

Target audience: Women who enjoy gardening (some men may enjoy this activity as well)

Objectives/outcomes:

- To provide a creative and expressive activity for interested residents

- To allow residents to express their creative ideas

- To promote residents' positive self-esteem through participation in successful projects

- To maintain and develop fine motor skills and hand-eye coordination

- To provide residents with opportunities to express choice and preference with regard to the finished product

- To provide mental stimulation, peer socialization, and recreation

- To provide for companionship and conversation

- To promote relaxation and communion with nature

- To provide an opportunity to nurture

- To provide a learning opportunity

Recommended group size: Small

Suggested time frame: One hour

Special needs/ability level (physical/cognitive skills needed): Any level of functioning with needed adaptations/simplifications

Activity outline:

- In the mid- to late winter, have the Garden Club select and plan what they want to plant in the garden area(s) by looking through garden catalogs; include flowers and vegetables. You may want to have someone from the Master Gardeners come and talk about gardening and conduct a planting demonstration during which the participants can get their hands in the dirt a little in the winter.

- In the early spring, have the Garden Club plant seeds for some of the garden plants and assist with watering and caring for the seedlings until planting season. If you have a greenhouse you can put the seedlings in there until they are ready to be planted outdoors.

- In the late spring, have the Garden Club transplant the seedlings and any purchased plants outdoors in the garden area(s).

- During the summer, have the Garden Club weed and water the garden area(s).

- All residents, family members, and staff members can enjoy the garden area(s) during the summer months by offering benches and walkways and encouraging people to utilize those areas. Encourage residents to pick and sample the garden tomatoes and cucumbers fresh from the vines. Allow the Cooking Club to use them also.

- If you have a greenhouse, plant some plants to stay in the greenhouse throughout the summer (e.g., tomatoes, peppers, and herbs do well inside a hot greenhouse).

- Have the Garden Club plan and fundraise for other additions to the garden area(s) (e.g., a water fountain, wind chimes, statuary, garden flags, bird houses, bird baths, etc.).

- Allow the Cooking Club to use any herbs that are grown.

Variations/adaptations/modifications: You will need to simplify tasks, make adaptations (provide raised garden beds, built-up gardening tools for participants with arthritic hands or for those who have difficulty grasping, and additional verbal and visual cues for lower-functioning residents), and give simpler tasks and offer more assistance to residents with diminished abilities, as they may be able to perform tasks with direct hand-over-hand guidance. Some activities can include low-functioning residents when adaptations/modifications are made. In-room, simple gardening can be offered by setting up a cart to take from room to room (e.g., starting seeds, transplanting plants, arranging fresh-cut flowers, etc.).

Helpful hints/notes: Seek donations of gardening supplies from garden centers and discount stores. Many are more than happy to donate or give reduced rates, especially at the end of the season, if you are not too fussy about what you want. Be sure to thank them and give them some free advertising as well. Much of the setup for these activities can be done prior to gathering residents so that you are ready to begin once residents have gathered. Assemble all needed equipment and supplies prior to the start of each activity.

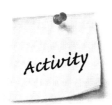

Activity   **Red Hat Society**

Target audience: Women's Club activity

Objectives/outcomes:

- Promotes social interaction between female peers and the staff

- Promotes camaraderie, a good time, sharing of stories, and (often) good food

- Provides an opportunity to "gossip" with the "girls"

- Provides for development of friendships, companionship, and conversation

- Provides an opportunity to meet other women with similar or varying interests

- Promotes reminiscence, mental stimulation, long-term memory skills, and cognitive/ thinking skills

- Provides a learning opportunity

- Provides an opportunity for recognition and to feel special (after all, what woman doesn't like special attention?)

Recommended group size: Small to medium

Suggested time frame: One hour

Special needs/ability level (physical/cognitive skills needed): Primarily residents with moderate to high cognitive functioning. Ability to reminisce, respond verbally, interact on some level, and complete tasks.

Activity outline:

- Hold the Red Hat Society club at least monthly. Have the Red Hat members decide what they will do each month. (Your January get-together can be to map out the monthly activities for the year.)

- Here's a little history of the Red Hat Society. "It all started as a result of a few women deciding to greet middle age with verve, humor, and élan," and was started by Sue

Ellen Cooper, Queen Mother, and her gifts to a few friends and the resulting "Red Hat Society" that formed. Sue Ellen's fondest hope is that these societies will proliferate far and wide. The main goal of the group is to have fun! It's seen as an opportunity for women who have shouldered responsibilities their whole lives to say goodbye to burdensome responsibilities and obligations for a while. It prides itself on "disorganization" by having no rules or bylaws to govern it. The only inflexible guidelines are that you must be a woman over the age of 50 (you're a Pink Hatter if you're under 50) and you must attend functions in full regalia (a red hat and purple outfit for women 50 and over, or a pink hat and lavender outfit for women under 50). You will also need to establish who the Chapter Queen is. Visit the official Red Hat Society Web site, *www.redhatsociety.com*, for additional information and to officially register your Red Hat Society group. It is strongly recommended that you register your group to make it official as this gives the group an air of importance and sophistication (the fee is nominal for a one-year membership).

- You will need to establish your Red Hat members and provide a name that fits your group.

- Have red hats available for the ladies to wear or encourage them to purchase their own. Have matching Red Hat T-shirts or have the ladies dress in red and purple for the gatherings. Encourage the women to wear any Red Hat paraphernalia.

- Some successful ideas include dining out, special luncheons, bus rides or trips, bingo, card games, picnics, cookouts, going shopping, visiting a greenhouse, hosting activities for other residents, being in a float for a community parade, inviting the Master Gardeners to do a demonstration, inviting the mayor (or other dignitary) to a special luncheon, meeting jointly with the Romeos a couple of times per year for socials, inviting community Red Hat Society groups to visit the facility for a joint activity, taking part in joint community Red Hat Society events, and virtually any activity that a Women's Club would enjoy.

Variations/adaptations/modifications: You may want to assign a female volunteer to oversee the club (to be the Queen Mother of the group), or you can have a staff member or resident fulfill this role. Solicit an organization to sponsor your group (e.g., a community women's club) to offset the cost of membership and associated costs for events held or attended.

Helpful hints/notes: Much of the setup for Red Hat Society events can be done prior to gathering residents so that you are ready to begin once residents have gathered. Assemble all needed equipment and supplies prior to the start of each activity. Observe all infection-control guidelines and individual resident dietary needs/restrictions when serving food and beverages.

Scrapbooking

Target audience: Women who enjoy crafts and helping others

Objectives/outcomes:

- To provide a creative and expressive activity for interested residents

- To allow residents to express their creative ideas

- To promote residents' positive self-esteem through participation in successful projects

- To maintain and develop fine motor skills and hand-eye coordination

- To provide residents with opportunities to express choice and preference with regard to the finished product

- To provide mental stimulation, peer socialization, and recreation

- To provide for companionship and conversation

- To promote relaxation

- To provide a learning opportunity and recognition

- To provide an opportunity to reminisce

Recommended group size: Small to medium (keep your staff-to-participant ratio manageable based on the amount of assistance needed by participants)

Suggested time frame: One hour

Special needs/ability level (physical/cognitive skills needed): Hand dexterity, ability to complete tasks, and creative ability

Activity outline:

- Purchase and have on hand a variety of scrapbook supplies. Supplies can be purchased individually or in kits. Supplies include a scrapbook, scrapbook pages, scrapbook papers, stamps, inks, stickers, pairs of scissors with different variegated edges, a scrapbook paper cutter, etc.

- This is a great way to get those activity pictures organized into books instead of left in boxes and drawers, never to see the light of day again, while simultaneously providing a great, creative activity for participants. Leaving completed scrapbooks displayed in activity areas for others to peruse at their pleasure will further advertise your activity programs; hence, this serves as an independent activity over and over.

- Provide each participant with needed supplies and a group of pictures that are similar in nature (e.g., pictures of the Senior Winter Olympics) so that your finished scrapbook is completed with some semblance of order. You do not want your finished scrapbook to be hodge-podge with no rhyme or reason (i.e., pictures of different events all mixed together). You want the participants to take a sense of pride in their work. Have each participant work on her individual page(s) to complete in the session, and at the end of the session put the pages into the book.

- Offer any individual assistance to participants as requested or needed, but allow them to express their own creativity.

- Document credit somewhere in the book for participants who assisted on the project to give them recognition (unless they choose not to be recognized).

- This can be an ongoing project scheduled routinely as you have enough pictures for a group of participants to work on. In this manner, the facility photos can be kept up-to-date, and participants can enjoy seeing themselves and their peers having a good time and can reminisce about the activity all over again.

Variations/adaptations/modifications: You will need to simplify tasks, make adaptations, provide built-up crafts tools for participants with arthritic hands or for those who have difficulty grasping, and additional verbal and visual cues for lower-functioning residents, and give simpler tasks and offer more assistance to residents with diminished abilities as they may be able to perform tasks with direct hand-over-hand guidance. Some activities can include low-functioning residents when adaptations/modifications are made. You also can provide participants with supplies in their rooms so that they can do some simple scrapbooking independently or with a staff member's help. Another variation is to schedule a family/resident scrapbooking activity whereby you contact the family of a participant, encouraging them to gather meaningful photos of their loved one throughout her life, and asking the family member(s) bring in all the supplies the resident will need for the activity (provide the family member[s] with a list of suggested supplies to bring). Then the family member(s) and the resident can create a scrapbook (life review book) together. The participants would keep their individual scrapbooks in their rooms for independent activity once completed. It may take several sessions, or you could conduct the initial get-started session and families and participants could complete the activity on their own as part of what they do when they come to visit, until it is completed. (They could also continue to add pages to it for an ongoing meaningful activity to share together.)

Helpful hints/notes: Purchase scrapbooking supplies from discount stores or when they go on clearance, as supplies can be quite costly. Monitor residents for safety when they're using scissors and paper cutters. Much of the setup for this activity can be done prior to gathering residents so that you are ready to begin once residents have gathered. Assemble all needed equipment and supplies prior to the start of the activity.

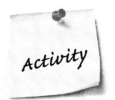 **Activity** | **Spa Day**

Target audience: Women who like to be pampered

Objectives/outcomes:

- Promotes social interaction between peers and the staff

- Provides for companionship and conversation

- Promotes relaxation

- Promotes self-esteem with pampering

- Provides a learning opportunity

Recommended group size: One-on-one within a small to medium-size group (participants can flow in and out throughout the day to give everyone who is interested a chance to take part)

Suggested time frame: 15 – 30 minutes, or up to one hour if a participant visits all stations, or as needed

Special needs/ability level (physical/cognitive skills needed): Primarily residents with moderate to high cognitive functioning

Activity outline:

- Set up the activity room/craft room/beauty shop or some private area to hold your spa.

- Set up stations in the room (e.g., manicure station, facial station, makeup station, massage station, etc.), with all needed supplies at each station. You will need washcloths and hand towels or disposable facial towels, facial mask/lotion, makeup (mainly powder/foundation, blush, and lipstick [use Q-tips and disposable makeup applicators to apply makeup for infection control purposes]), nail polish (in a variety of colors) and nail polish remover, disposable emery boards (one per participant), and scented hand/body lotion for massages (a gentle massage of the face, shoulders, and upper back and a hand massage are options that can be offered). Another option is to use a gentle exfoliating sugar hand scrub, followed by massage and scented lotion. (This will require a sink area for running water or a basin with water that is sanitized between participants.) Staff members and volunteers will need to wash their hands after working with each participant.

- Use a soothing aromatherapy scent in a diffuser (e.g., lavender or vanilla).

- Play relaxing background music (e.g., instrumental or classical) and have subdued lighting. A tabletop water fountain is another nice relaxing option.

- Have participants go around to the stations that are of interest to them. Some will want to visit each station and others will be interested in only some stations. A staff member or volunteer will need to man each station. Have the participants move through the stations in the natural order: starting with the massage station (preparing face and hands and getting participants in a relaxed state), then the facial station, then the manicure station (can get this done while the mask is on the face), and ending with the makeup station.

- Have healthy snacks and drinks for the participants to sample once they have gone around to all the stations they are interested in (granola bars, fresh fruit, and vegetable and natural fruit juices are good healthy options), and promote socialization with others.

- Advertise your event ahead of time with special posters.

Variations/adaptations/modifications: You could have a "spa cart" that goes from room to room for those who are unable or unwilling to come down to a group setting. You can also have a manicure cart go from room to room.

Helpful hints/notes: Seek donations of makeup from Avon or Mary Kay demonstrators. Much of the setup for this event can be done prior to gathering residents so that you are ready to begin once residents have gathered. Assemble all needed equipment and supplies prior to the start of the activity. Observe all infection-control guidelines and individual resident dietary needs/restrictions when serving food and beverages.

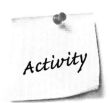 *Activity*

Tea Social/Gourmet Coffee Social

Target audience: Women's Club activity

Objectives/outcomes:

- Promotes social interaction between female peers and the staff

- Promotes camaraderie, a good time, sharing of stories, and good food

- Provides an opportunity to "gossip" with the "girls"

- Provides for development of friendships, companionship, and conversation

- Provides an opportunity to meet other women with similar or varying interests

- Promotes reminiscence

Recommended group size: Small to medium

Suggested time frame: One hour, or as needed

Special needs/ability level (physical/cognitive skills needed): Primarily residents with moderate to high cognitive functioning

Activity outline:

- Schedule a tea social just for women.

- Have on hand a variety of teas (herbal, black, green, decaffeinated) so that participants have a choice.

- Use teacups and saucers to make it a fancy tea gathering. You can purchase these from rummage sales, Good Will, or secondhand stores, or seek donations of mismatched sets, which can promote some interesting conversation.

- Serve teacakes, scones, biscotti, and small, fancy gourmet cookies. (Make them ahead of time, purchase them from a bakery, or secure them through your Dietary Department.)

- Promote conversation throughout.

- Play quiet background music to set the mood.

Variations/adaptations/modifications: Instead of a tea social, have a gourmet coffee social. For this you would provide a variety of gourmet coffees (serve instant coffee or you can select one gourmet coffee bean and make one flavor in a drip coffeemaker). Instead of tea-cups, serve in coffee mugs with handles (discourage the use of paper or foam cups for safety, environmental, and aesthetic reasons; you want this to be a special social and paper products just don't cut it).

Helpful hints/notes: Much of the setup for this event can be done prior to gathering residents so that you are ready to begin once residents have gathered. Assemble all needed equipment and supplies prior to the start of the activity. Observe all infection-control guidelines and individual resident dietary needs/restrictions when serving food and beverages.

Chapter 9

Activities for Bariatric Residents

Obesity is a rising medical problem. Obesity is associated with many detrimental health problems: heart disease, diabetes, many forms of cancer, asthma, obstructive sleep apnea, and chronic musculoskeletal problems, among others. Obesity also has a clear effect on mortality. Bariatrics is the branch of medicine that deals with the causes, prevention, and treatment of obesity.

The Body Mass Index is widely adopted and promoted as a marker for excess body weight, but it is not flawless. Waist circumference and a person's risk factors for diseases and conditions associated with obesity are other markers for the evaluation of obesity.

Diet, exercise, behavior therapy, and anti-obesity drugs are the first-line treatments. These therapies, however, have limited short-term success and nearly nonexistent long-term success. Bariatric surgery has been the popular treatment for obesity. This generally results in greater weight loss than conventional treatment and improves quality of life by reducing obesity-related diseases. One of the most rewarding aspects of bariatric surgery is the transformation of health and the increase in quality of life that many patients experience. Bariatric surgery patients sometimes experience complications as a result of the surgery. These include gastrointestinal symptoms including vomiting, diarrhea, dysphagia, and reflux; anastomotic leaking at the surgical connections between the stomach and the intestine; abdominal hernia requiring further surgery; and infections.

Recovery takes time and patience. The diet is strict and progressive, and patients usually have pain while they heal. Getting enough protein and nutrients is critical for the rest of a bariatric resident's life span.

The treatment requires permanent lifestyle changes once the surgery is complete. This means residents need to develop healthy habits for both diet and fitness, something most did not have prior to the surgery, though it is recommended that residents begin this prior to surgery. Regular exercise, next to following the bariatric program's dietary guidelines, is an important factor when it comes to optimizing health outcomes and quality of life after bariatric surgery. Initial exercises are walking and doing other leg exercises as soon as possible after surgery. This helps residents avoid deep vein thrombosis. Bariatric residents should phase in exercise as soon after surgery as possible. Walking for at least five minutes five days per week is a great introduction to exercising, because it is low-impact; residents are then advised to gradually increase the amount of time they spend exercising by adding a few minutes each week.

Another important aspect of treatment is emotional health as the road to recovery is a long journey with ups and downs. It is not uncommon for some residents to experience a period of "postoperative blues" during the first weeks after bariatric surgery. This often occurs when residents start to feel better, but before they experience a return in energy and stamina. They may even second-guess their decision to have surgery. This is usually only temporary. An important part of ongoing care is participation in a support group where experiences can be shared among others going through the same thing; experiences which family and friends may not understand. Having a support network is essential in ensuring success.

Not all bariatric residents will comply with these lifestyle changes. Remember that they have lived their entire lives with these established bad habits, and family members may have knowingly or unknowingly enabled them in their ways. It is difficult to change a long-established habit, especially if the resident lacks desire and motivation for making necessary lifestyle changes to achieve positive results.

There may be other barriers to pursuing leisure interests, such as mobility impairments, embarrassment related to obesity, shortness of breath with exertion, inability to tolerate being up for prolonged periods, and general lack of energy and stamina. The care planning team needs to address all of these on an individual basis.

With these things in mind, activities professionals need to work with the therapy department, nursing department, social services, physician, mental health professional, and dietitian in developing a comprehensive care plan to meet the unique needs of bariatric residents. Activities professionals can be an element of support and can coordinate activities that promote a healthier lifestyle by offering cooking classes on healthy cooking; serving healthy snack options at activities; setting up an exercise program that is progressive as the residents gains strength and mobility; and assisting in making sure the patient gets to scheduled support groups as desired. Activities professionals should also encourage and assist as needed with assessed individual leisure interests, whether they involve independent, one-on-one, or group activities.

Use the following activities to enhance programming for bariatric residents. Note that many bariatric residents are younger than traditional nursing home residents and their needs, abilities, and interests can vary widely. Activities professionals need to adapt their programming to fit each individual bariatric resident.

Bariatric Ball Exercise

Target audience: Bariatric residents

Objectives/outcomes:

- To build staff and resident rapport

- To provide an opportunity for socialization

- To enhance therapy goals

- To promote a healthy lifestyle

- To improve balance and reduce the risk of falls

- To improve mobility and function

- To improve coordination

- To improve cardiovascular endurance

- To improve mind-body coordination

- To decrease joint pain

- To alleviate chronic pain

- To improve sleep

- To reduce stiffness

- To help prevent sarcopenia (progressive muscle loss)

- To help prevent bone loss

- To improve blood pressure and circulation

- To decrease depression

- To improve cognition and short-term memory

- To enhance vitality and energy

- To promote weight loss

- To provide a learning opportunity

- To promote a healthy lifestyle and formation of healthy habits

- To build strength and endurance and help residents regain their independence

Recommended group size: Independent, one-on-one, or any size group

Suggested time frame: Will vary according to ability, but should be progressive, adding more time each week

Special needs/ability level (physical/cognitive skills needed): Individuals who can sit on the exercise ball and follow actions and physically complete a series of movements. An appropriate individual program needs to be devised for each participant, taking into account his or her health status and abilities.

Activity outline:

- Work in conjunction with the therapy department on individual participant goals.

- You will need a large exercise ball for each participant. (This would typically be appropriate for a younger bariatric resident.)

- Here are some sample exercises:

  - Pelvic tilt: Sit on the ball and gently roll forward and backward. Repeat 10 times per set.

  - Lateral pelvic tilt: Sit on the ball and gently move your hips from side to side. Repeat 10 times per set.

  - Pelvic circles: Sit on the ball and rotate your pelvis clockwise 10 times, and then counterclockwise 10 times.

  - Sitting bilateral shoulder flexion: Sit on the ball and raise your arms over your head, and then lower them. Repeat 10 times per set.

  - Sitting bilateral arm abduction: Raise your arms out to the side and lower them. Repeat 10 times.

  - Forward sitting flex and extension: Sit forward on the ball. Raise one arm across your body and above your head, following the movement of your arm with your head and leaning back slightly while reaching. Repeat on the other side. Repeat 10 times on both sides.

– Kneeling neck extension: Lie on your stomach over the ball and let your back stretch. Hold for 30 – 60 seconds. Repeat 10 times.

– Prone alternating arm raise: Laying over the ball with hands and toes touching the floor, raise one arm and return. Repeat with the other arm. Repeat 10 times for each arm.

– Kneeling side-to-side stretch: From a kneeling position, stretch to one side, rolling the ball with you. Hold for five seconds and repeat on the other side. Repeat 10 times per side.

– Bridging with arm raise: In a bridging position (lie on the ball with your upper shoulders resting on the ball and your knees bent and your feet flat on the floor), raise one arm over your head and parallel to the floor. Maintain your balance. Repeat with the other arm. Repeat 10 times with both arms.

• Praise everyone's efforts.

• Provide a copy of this exercise to bariatric residents upon discharge.

Variations/adaptations/modifications: You will need to know the individual abilities of residents and provide any needed modifications. Provide verbal and visual cues. Simplify movements as needed. One variation involves some simple stretching exercises, which you can do on a bed or mat:

• Pelvic tilt: Lie on your back and flatten your back by tightening your stomach muscles and buttocks. Repeat 10 – 20 times per set.

• Trunk stability: Lie on your back with a pillow behind your head, and with your knees off the bed/mat and your feet flat on the bed/mat. Tighten your stomach and slowly slide your foot on the bed/mat until your leg is nearly straight, but do not let your back begin to arch. Repeat with the other leg. Repeat 10 – 20 times per set.

• Lie on your back and tighten your stomach muscles. Slowly raise one leg off the bed/floor and lower it back down. Keep your back flat on the bed/floor and your stomach tight. Repeat with your other leg. Repeat 10 – 20 times per set.

- Lie flat, with your knees bent and your feet flat on the bed/floor and your arms above your head. Tighten your stomach and slowly raise one leg and lower the opposite arm from over your head down to your side. Keep your stomach tight and back flat. Return to the starting position. Repeat with the opposite side. Repeat 10 – 20 times per set.

- Lie on your back with your knees bent and your feet flat on the bed/floor. Slowly raise your buttocks from the bed/floor, keeping your stomach tight. Return to the starting position. Repeat 10 – 20 times per set.

- Lower trunk rotation stretch: Lie on your back, with your knees bent and your feet together and flat on the bed/floor. Keep your back flat and your feet together and rotate your knees to each side. Hold for five seconds per side, or 10 times total.

- Knee-to-chest stretch: Lie on your back, place your hands behind your knees, and pull both knees into your chest until you can feel a comfortable stretch in your lower back and buttocks. Stay relaxed. Hold for 30 seconds. Repeat three times per set.

- Mid-back rotation stretch: Sit upright on your bed/floor with your legs spread out as far as you can. Reach to each side as far as possible, keeping your chest low to the floor. Hold for 30 seconds. Repeat two times in each direction.

- Angry cat stretch: Get on all fours on the floor or the bed, tuck your chin and tighten your stomach, arching your back. Repeat 10 times per set.

Helpful hints/notes: Advertise and promote these activities for bariatric residents. Consult with the physician to ensure appropriateness for each individual bariatric residents and to ensure that he or she can participate safely in the activity. Have participants wear comfortable shoes and clothing. Make sure participants drink plenty of water and take frequent breaks.

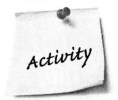

Bariatric Cooking Class

Target audience: Bariatric residents

Objectives/outcomes:

- Promotes social interaction between peers and the staff

- Provides for development of friendships, companionship, and conversation

- Promotes reminiscence, mental stimulation, long-term memory skills, and cognitive/ thinking skills

- Promotes creative expression and choice

- Promotes weight loss

- Provides a learning opportunity

- Promotes a healthy lifestyle and formation of healthy habits

Recommended group size: Small to medium (12 – 15)

Suggested time frame: One hour, or as needed

Special needs/ability level (physical/cognitive skills needed): Primarily residents with moderate to high cognitive functioning

Activity outline:

- Hold this activity weekly (you may want to work in conjunction with the Occupational Therapy department).

- Have participants look through special recipes/books. Try a variety of healthy recipes that are low in sugar, fat, and processed grains and are high in protein, fiber, and nutrient density. One caveat: The participants must be able to complete and serve the recipe in the time allotted for the activity. As an alternative, participants can make the recipe in the morning and serve it at an afternoon activity.

- Either shop for or secure needed items from the Dietary Department.

- Have all residents wash their hands prior to preparing food.

- Follow and prepare the recipe, dividing the tasks (cleaning, chopping, cutting, measuring, stirring, etc.) among individual participants so that they all have tasks that they are capable of completing.

- Discuss healthy eating habits while the food cooks/bakes.

- Sample the recipe when complete.

- Serve a beverage as well.

- Promote conversation throughout.

- Give copies of recipes to bariatric patients upon discharge.

Variations/adaptations/modifications: You will need to simplify tasks, make adaptations (provide built-up utensils, special cutting boards that hold items in place for those with use of only one arm/hand, and additional verbal and visual cues for lower-functioning residents), and give simpler tasks and offer more assistance to residents with diminished abilities as they may be able to perform tasks with direct hand-over-hand guidance. Some activities can include low-functioning residents when adaptations/modifications are made.

Helpful hints/notes: Make sure participants use caution with sharp knives, and do not leave participants unsupervised. Much of the setup for this activity can be done prior to gathering residents so that you are ready to begin once residents have gathered. Assemble all needed equipment and supplies prior to the start of the activity. Observe all infection-control guidelines and individual resident dietary needs/restrictions when serving food and beverages.

Sample Recipes:

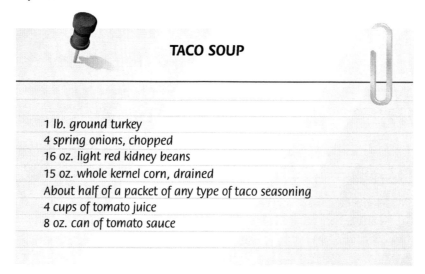

TACO SOUP

1 lb. ground turkey
4 spring onions, chopped
16 oz. light red kidney beans
15 oz. whole kernel corn, drained
About half of a packet of any type of taco seasoning
4 cups of tomato juice
8 oz. can of tomato sauce

Sauté and brown the turkey with the chopped onions for about seven minutes. Remove from heat and drain. Place drained meat mixture into a large saucepan and add remaining ingredients. Heat thoroughly, but do not boil! Serves six. 225 calories per serving, 21 grams protein.

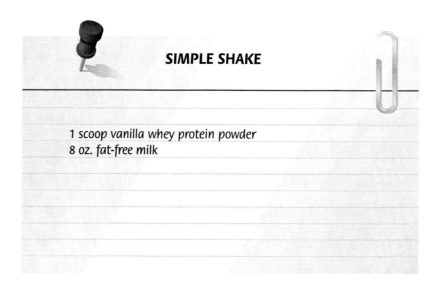

SIMPLE SHAKE

1 scoop vanilla whey protein powder
8 oz. fat-free milk

Mix well in a shaker cup or blender. 28 grams protein.

Variation: Add one scoop (individual serving) sugar-free Sunrise Orange Crystal Light powder to make an Orange Dreamsicle.

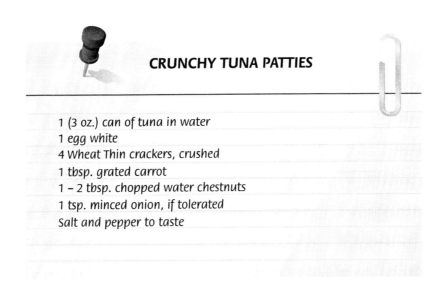

CRUNCHY TUNA PATTIES

1 (3 oz.) can of tuna in water
1 egg white
4 Wheat Thin crackers, crushed
1 tbsp. grated carrot
1 – 2 tbsp. chopped water chestnuts
1 tsp. minced onion, if tolerated
Salt and pepper to taste

Mix all ingredients together. Spray medium-size skillet with nonstick cooking spray. Cook patties until golden brown. Serves two. 80 calories per serving, and 12 grams protein.

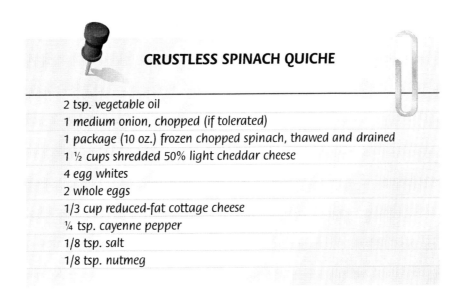

CRUSTLESS SPINACH QUICHE

2 tsp. vegetable oil
1 medium onion, chopped (if tolerated)
1 package (10 oz.) frozen chopped spinach, thawed and drained
1 ½ cups shredded 50% light cheddar cheese
4 egg whites
2 whole eggs
1/3 cup reduced-fat cottage cheese
¼ tsp. cayenne pepper
1/8 tsp. salt
1/8 tsp. nutmeg

Heat oven to 375°F. Coat a 9-inch pie pan with vegetable oil spray. In a medium-size non-stick skillet, heat oil on medium-high. Add onion and cook five minutes or until softened. Add spinach and stir three more minutes, or until spinach is dry; set aside. Sprinkle cheese in pie pan. Top with spinach/onion mixture. In medium bowl, whisk egg whites and whole eggs, cottage cheese, cayenne pepper, salt, and nutmeg. Pour mixture over spinach. Bake 30 – 35 minutes or until set. Let stand five minutes. Cut into wedges and serve. Serves four. 231 calories per serving, and 24 grams protein.

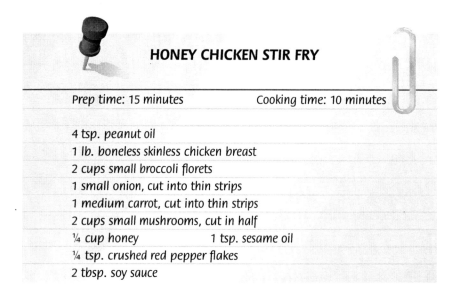

HONEY CHICKEN STIR FRY

Prep time: 15 minutes   Cooking time: 10 minutes

4 tsp. peanut oil
1 lb. boneless skinless chicken breast
2 cups small broccoli florets
1 small onion, cut into thin strips
1 medium carrot, cut into thin strips
2 cups small mushrooms, cut in half
¼ cup honey   1 tsp. sesame oil
¼ tsp. crushed red pepper flakes
2 tbsp. soy sauce

In a large skillet, heat oil over medium-high heat; add chicken and sauté for three minutes. Add the broccoli, onion, carrot, and mushrooms and sauté for five minutes. Add the honey, sesame oil, red pepper flakes, and soy sauce. Stir until all vegetables are glazed and sauce is bubbly hot, about one minute. Serve. Serves six.

Tip: Make sure all the pieces of chicken are the same size so that they will cook evenly. Variation: You can use shrimp and scallops in the recipe instead of chicken. 181 calories per serving, and 18 grams protein.

SALMON BLUSH

Prep time: 5 minutes   Cooking time: 12 minutes
Serves four
1 tbsp. butter
2 tbsp. olive oil
1 lb. salmon fillets
1 tsp. garlic, chopped
2 tbsp. capers
¼ cup red wine
¼ cup heavy cream
Salt and pepper to taste
1 tbsp. fresh parsley

In a large sauté pan over medium-high heat, add butter and olive oil. When butter and oil are heated, add the salmon. Sauté for 5 – 8 minutes, depending on the thickness of the salmon, turning the salmon over every two minutes. Add the garlic, capers, wine, and cream. Bring to a simmer and let simmer for four minutes. Add the salt, pepper, and parsley. Serve.

Variation: You can use other fish such as grouper, sea bass, or mahi-mahi in this recipe for a change of pace. Serves four. 343 calories per serving, and 26 grams protein.

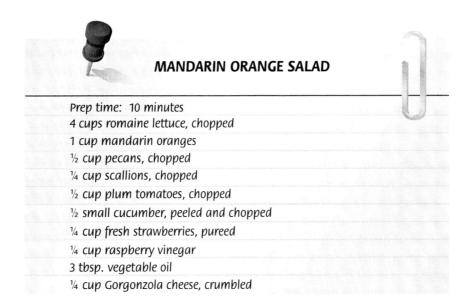

MANDARIN ORANGE SALAD

Prep time: 10 minutes
4 cups romaine lettuce, chopped
1 cup mandarin oranges
½ cup pecans, chopped
¼ cup scallions, chopped
½ cup plum tomatoes, chopped
½ small cucumber, peeled and chopped
¼ cup fresh strawberries, pureed
¼ cup raspberry vinegar
3 tbsp. vegetable oil
¼ cup Gorgonzola cheese, crumbled

Place all ingredients in a large bowl and mix well. Serve. Serves eight. 253 calories per serving, and 4 grams protein.

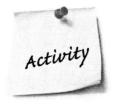

Bariatric Exercise

Target audience: Bariatric residents

Objectives/outcomes:

- To build staff and resident rapport

- To provide an opportunity for socialization

- To enhance therapy goals

- To promote a healthy lifestyle

- To improve balance and reduce the risk of falls

- To improve mobility and function

- To improve coordination

- To improve cardiovascular endurance

- To improve mind-body coordination

- To decrease joint pain

- To alleviate chronic pain

- To improve sleep

- To reduce stiffness

- To help prevent sarcopenia (progressive muscle loss)

- To help prevent bone loss

- To improve blood pressure and circulation

- To decrease depression

- To improve cognition and short-term memory

- To enhance vitality and energy

- To promote weight loss

- To provide a learning opportunity

- To promote a healthy lifestyle and formation of healthy habits

- To build strength and endurance and help residents regain their independence

Recommended group size: Independent, one-on-one, or any size group

Suggested time frame: Will vary according to ability, but should be progressive, adding more time each week

Special needs/ability level (physical/cognitive skills needed): Individuals who can follow actions and physically complete a series of movements. An appropriate individual program needs to be devised for each participant, taking into account his or her health status and abilities.

Activity outline:

- Work in conjunction with the therapy department on individual participant goals. Some movements are more appropriate for younger bariatric residents.

- Begin with warm-ups. Any one of the following is acceptable: walking at a casual pace for five minutes, marching in place, stationary bicycling, shrugging shoulders up and down, swinging arms, or doing leg lifts.

- Stretching (warms up the muscles): Yoga and tai chi moves are great stretching exercises (see Chapter 6). Other stretching movements include raising your arms above your head and stretching; sitting on a chair with your legs out in front of you and raising your legs and stretching; and putting your arms out to your sides and stretching first the left arm and then the right.

- Aerobic activity (gets the heart rate up): You can choose from walking (increasing the speed and distance as fitness improves), swimming, water aerobics, cardio kickboxing (see the discussion on martial arts in Chapter 6), stair-climbing, jogging, using an elliptical machine, bicycling, spinning classes, rowing machines, and DVD and video exercises. Choose from these options depending on availability and on each participant's ability level.

- Strength training (builds muscle mass): This involves using resistance bands and weights (see Chapter 6 for additional exercise examples). Here are some sample moves using resistance bands or resistance cords (these are advanced moves requiring mat work; some moves can be adapted to a sitting chair position):

    - Zip up: Stand and grasp the handles of the cord or ends of the band in each hand. Gently step on the center of the cord/band. Rest your palms on your thighs, with the ends touching. Now, inhale and keep the handles/ends close to your body and pull along the centerline of your body to your upper chest, as though you are zipping up a zipper. Bend your elbows at your sides, not in front of you. Exhale and slowly lower your arms and hands or the cords back to the original position, resisting as you go.

    - Chest expansion: Stand and grasp the handles/ends of the cord/band in each hand, and gently step on the center. Let your arms hang long at your sides, palms facing back, and thumbs touching your outer thighs. Squeeze your shoulder blades together to open your chest. Pull your shoulders away from your ears. Keep your arms straight, inhale, and press your palms straight back, bringing your shoulder blades together. Hold your breath as you turn your head slowly to the left and then to the right, stretching your neck and shoulder muscles. Return your head to the center and exhale as you release your arms back down to your sides.

    - Arm circles: Kneel on the middle of the cord/band and sit back on your heels. The band or cord should be under your shins. Your ankles, knees, and inner thighs should be touching each other. Squeeze your shoulder blades together. Pull your navel toward your spine. Grasp each handle/end of the cord/band and bring your arms straight out in front of your chest, palms facing down and arms parallel to the floor. Inhale through your nose and begin making small, controlled circles with your arms, beginning by circling each arm out and away from your body. Circle your entire arm from the shoulder to the joint. Exhale and reverse the circles.

    - Biceps curl: Hold on to each handle/end of the cord/band and stand on the center of the cord/band with your arms long by your sides, palms facing forward. Pull your navel toward your spine. Squeeze your shoulder blades together and pull your shoulders down. Keep your elbows glued to the sides of your body. Inhale and slowly curl your arms in front of your body, palms and forearms in toward your shoulders. Exhale and slowly uncurl your arms back to the starting position.

- Standing shoulder stretches: Stand with your feet parallel and hip-width apart. Fold the cord/band in half and hold it with both hands. Your hands should be shoulder-width apart and your palms should be facing down. Bring the cord/band in front of you to shoulder level. Now inhale, pull your navel in toward your spine, lift your arms, and bring the cord/band back behind you as far as you can go. Stretch the cord/band out as much as you can and keep your torso in line with your hips. Now inhale and bring the cord/band forward and over your head. Exhale and return your arms and the cord/band back in front of you to the starting position.

- Here are some sample moves using hand weights (begin with light weights and increase the weight as fitness improves; moves can be done from a sitting or standing position). Either stand straight or sit straight, maintaining good posture throughout the exercise sequence. Repeat the exercise sequences, adding repetitions as fitness improves.

  - Grasp a weight in both hands (or in one hand) and hold it down at your sides, palms facing forward. Slowly raise your hands, bending at the elbows, to waist position. Now place your hands down at your sides with your palms facing the sides. Slowly raise your arms straight out to your sides. Return to the starting position.

  - Holding the weights in your hands, hold your arms directly out in front of you, palms up. Slowly bend your elbows toward your shoulders and return to the starting position.

  - Hold the weights in both hands in front of you, with your elbows bent and your palms facing you. Slowly raise one hand above your head while you simultaneously lower your other hand to your side. Bring your arm back to the starting position and reverse the movement.

  - Holding the weights in your hands with your elbows bent and your palms facing toward your face slowly raise your arms above your head as high as you can. Return to the starting position.

- Always end the exercise session with a cool-down and stretches. Deep breathing exercises should be included as well.

- Praise everyone's efforts.

- Provide a copy of these exercises to bariatric patients at discharge.

Variations/adaptations/modifications: Residents who sit in wheelchairs can perform some of these actions from a sitting position with a leader's help. You will need to know the individual abilities of residents and provide the needed modifications. Provide verbal and visual cues. Simplify movements as needed.

Helpful hints/notes: Advertise and promote this activity to bariatric residents. Consult with the physician to ensure appropriateness for each individual bariatric resident and to ensure that he or she can participate safely in the activity. Have participants wear comfortable shoes and clothing. Make sure participants drink plenty of water and take frequent breaks.

Chapter 10

One-on-One Activities

One-on-one activities are an important part of any activity program. They are required for residents who are unable to participate in groups, for residents who decline or refuse to participate in groups, and as a supplement to group programming to meet the individual leisure interests of all residents. The Centers for Medicare & Medicaid Services defines one-on-one programming as "programming provided to residents who will not or cannot effectively plan their own activity pursuits, or residents needing specialized or extended programs to enhance their overall daily routine and activity pursuits."

It is the facility's responsibility to provide one-on-one activities to residents; therefore, all staff members should be providing one-on-one activities to residents throughout the day. Certified nursing assistants can provide one-on-one activities during daily care and while assisting with meals by interacting with residents about things of interest to them. They can discuss the residents' families, talk about current events within the facility and/or community, and provide supportive reality orientation (RO)(e.g., weather, season, time of year, current/upcoming holidays, etc.). They can also paint a resident's fingernails, softly brush a resident's hair, apply lotion or give a simple hand massage to a resident, take a resident outdoors for a walk or just to sit in the sunshine, sing with a resident, read to a resident, set up a resident's favorite videos/DVDs, play a resident's favorite radio station or music CDs, play card or board games with a resident, set up a jigsaw puzzle or work with a resident on a jigsaw puzzle, do crosswords with a resident, set up a resident with manipulatives (all-in-one boards is one example)—whatever is of interest to the resident and what he or she is capable of doing. All other departments can provide positive social interactions, which will raise the resident's self-esteem, bring smiles, and make the resident feel good, all of which have a positive effect on the resident's quality of life. All staff members should be interacting with residents, even in passing (e.g., notice hair appointments, comment on how they look, comment on the day, reassure someone who is anxious, and provide residents with meaningful things to do).

To enable all staff members to provide activities the activities professionals must keep every unit/household well supplied with leisure interest materials pertinent to the residents who reside there. These materials need to be accessible to all staff members 24/7. Activities professionals also need to educate all staff members through yearly inservices about providing activities to residents.

Most activities that can be done in a group setting can be done or modified for use on a one-on-one basis, if the resident is interested in that activity but cannot or chooses not to be involved in a group. Some examples of one-on-one activities besides those mentioned earlier include:

- Sensory stimulation programs

- Cognitive therapy

- Reminiscence

- Support of self-directed activity of the resident's choosing (delivering supplies, setting up materials)

- Task-oriented activities

- Crafts

- Pet visits

- Word puzzles

- Trivia sheets

- Helping a resident to write a letter

- Helping a resident to use a computer, the Internet, or e-mail

- Bringing a Wii (or other electronic game console) into a resident's room so that he or she can play it

- Offering the use of handheld games

- Visiting a resident with the library cart

You can purchase many activity supplies specifically designed to provide various one-on-one activities. Because we have already addressed many one-on-one programs elsewhere in this book, in this chapter we provide only two additional examples.

Memories

Target audience: Residents who need or prefer one-on-one activities, or as a supplement to group programming

Objectives/outcomes:

- To promote communication and enjoyment

- To encourage interaction with others and increase social contact

- To enhance/increase attention span and memory recall, thinking, reasoning and concentration skills, and reminiscence

- To provide person-centered care and promote positive memories of a participant's past

Recommended group size: One-on-one

Suggested time frame: 10 minutes

Special needs/ability level (physical/cognitive skills needed): All levels

Activity outline:

- Select a topic or subject that is seasonal, themed, or of interest to the participant.

- This is a reminiscence activity, so bring relevant materials along on visits. These can include books, magazines, pictures and other visual props, scents—whatever will help to stimulate the resident's responses and ability to reminisce.

- Read to the resident, or have him or her read to you. Have the resident look at, touch, and hold any props. Ask simple, open-ended questions to promote responses/conversation. Begin questions with what, who, when, where, why, and how. Let the course of the discussion and length of the session be dictated by the participant's responses.

- Close the session with a positive comment and thank the resident for participating.

Variations/adaptations/modifications: You have to adapt/modify your approach based on the cognitive ability level of each individual. Provide the visual, verbal, and direct physical guidance that each person needs to be successful. Redirect as necessary. You will need to offer more assistance to residents with diminished abilities. This requires that you have assessed the abilities and identified the needs, interests, and interventions of each resident.

Helpful hints/notes: Have on hand a supply of material that will evoke reminiscence on a variety of subjects.

Morning Stretch

Target audience: Residents who need or prefer one-on-one activities, or as a supplement to group programming

Objectives/outcomes:

- To provide an opportunity for communication

- To promote large motor physical activity and enjoyment

- To encourage interaction with others and increase social contact

- To enhance/increase attention span and concentration and promote the ability to follow one-step directions or mimic desired actions

- To improve mood by actively engaging the resident at his or her level of ability

- To promote the ability of the participant to express him or herself

- To promote person-centered care

- To improve relationships between caregivers and residents

Recommended group size: One-on-one

Suggested time frame: 5 – 10 minutes

Special needs/ability level (physical/cognitive skills needed): Residents with the physical capacity to follow one-step directions or mimic desired actions

Activity outline:

- This should be scheduled in the morning, soon after breakfast. It is an activity to get the resident excited for the day by getting his or her blood flowing, announcing the day (e.g., activities for the day, the day's weather), and giving the resident something to look forward to.

- Announce and demonstrate the following simple stretching exercises, starting at the top of the body and working your way down:

– Head/neck: Turn your head to the left, then to the center, and then to the right. Look up and then down, touch your left ear to your left shoulder and then your right ear to your right shoulder, and rotate your neck.

– Shoulders: Shrug your shoulders up and down; roll your shoulders backward and forward.

– Arms: Hang your arms down at your sides and do small arm circles, first one way and then the other. Now put your arms out to your sides and make small circles in a forward motion, gradually making the circles bigger. Then make small circles in a backward motion, gradually making the circles bigger. Now place your arms out in front of you, palms up. Curl your arms up to your shoulders until they touch. Hold your arms out in front of you, palms facing down, and make wrist circles, first one way and then the other. End by opening and closing your fists.

– Legs: March in place, lifting your knees as high as possible. Put your feet flat on the floor, and raise one leg up and down and then the other leg up and down. Raise one foot off the floor and do ankle circles one way and then the other; repeat with the other foot. Finish by placing your feet flat on the floor and rocking your feet back and forth from heel to toe.

• Thank the resident for his or her participation.

Variations/adaptations/modifications: You have to adapt/modify your approach based on the physical and cognitive ability level of each individual. Provide the visual, verbal, and direct physical guidance that each person needs to be successful. Redirect as necessary. You will need to offer more assistance to residents with diminished abilities (they may be able to perform tasks with direct hand-over-hand guidance). This requires that you have assessed the abilities and identified the needs, interests, and interventions of each resident.

Helpful hints/notes: Encourage residents who are able to do this activity as part of their own morning routine.

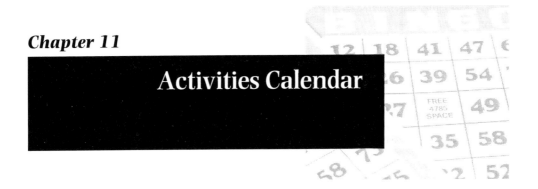

Chapter 11

Activities Calendar

The activities calendar is the formal activity program, or schedule of the events that are going to occur during a given month. Of course, as we've already discussed, besides the activities on the calendar, additional spontaneous activities should be occurring on a daily basis—for example, having ice cream cones on the patio during nice weather, among other individual and one-on-one activities.

The activities included on the activities calendar should occur as scheduled and on time. Rarely should an activity on the calendar be canceled (e.g., a musician can't come in because he or she is ill); if this occurs, a substitute activity should be offered.

The activities calendar needs to reflect the interests, needs, and abilities of the residents who reside in the facility. The program needs to be reviewed on an ongoing basis to ensure that these standards are being met. The calendar should include one-on-one, small-group, and large-group programming in a variety of areas to meet the social, spiritual, psychosocial, physical, mental/cognitive, and emotional needs of all residents.

The activities program should include activities that are seasonal, holiday-themed, cultural, religious, music-themed, recreational, social, creative, educational, and active/exercise-themed. It should also include outings, family events, special programs/events, outdoor events—in other words, it should include something for everyone and reflect resident interests.

In this chapter, we've provided two sample activities calendars: One is a general activities calendar and the other is an activities calendar for specialized programming for dementia residents. We've also included a sample calendar-planning list located on the CD-ROM, list so that you can keep an updated list of activity supplies on hand to help you plan your activities calendar.

APRIL 2008 ACTIVITY SCHEDULE OF EVENTS
PORTAGE COUNTY HEALTH CARE CENTER

ACTIVITIES DIRECTOR: DEBBIE BERA
ACTIVITIES ASSISTANTS: MIRA MELCHER(EAST/SOUTH) TERRY MILLER(NORTH)
TINA BERG(SOUTH)
SCHEDULE SUBJECT TO CHANGE/OBSERVE DAILY POSTINGS

CODE
SR = Sensory Room   DR = Dining Room
AA = Activity Area   E = East Wing
AK = Activity Kitchen   N = North Wing
AW = All Wings   S = South Wing
CH = Chapel   FR = Family Room
O = Outing

SUNDAY	MONDAY	TUESDAY	WEDNESDAY	THURSDAY	FRIDAY	SATURDAY
		1 National Fun at Work Day! April Fool's Day! 9:30 a.m. Ring Toss (AA) 10 a.m. Library Cart (AW) 10:45 a.m. Morning Glory Chapel (CH) 2 p.m. Shake Loose a Memory (AK) 2 p.m. Romeos – Chicken Shoot (AA) 3:30 p.m. One-on-One Therapeutic Massage (AW)	**2** 9 a.m. Memories (AW) 9:45 a.m. Friends & Fellowship (CH) **10:15 a.m. Food Committee (DR)** 11:45 a.m. Stretchercize (DR) 1:30 p.m. Rosary (CH) 2 p.m. Catholic Mass (CH) **2:30 p.m. Music w/David, Chet & Gang (AA)** 6 p.m. Card Club (AA)	**3** 9:15 a.m. Sunshine Group (AK) **9:30 a.m. Disc Golf w/students (AA)** 10:30 a.m. Church of the Intercession and Holy Communion (CH) 2 p.m. Music w/Gene Hersey (AA) 3:30 p.m. One-on-One Room Visit (AW)	**4** 9 a.m. Morning Greeting (N) 10 a.m. Pilates (AA) 10:30 a.m. Out to Lunch Bunch (O) **1:30 p.m. CDA Bingo (DR)** 3:30 p.m. One-on-One Room Visits (AW) 4:30 p.m. Music w/Marilyn Pederson (AA)	**5** Weekend Trivia (AW) 9 a.m. Morning Stretch (AW) 10 a.m. Busy Bee Crafts (AK) 10 a.m. Pet Therapy w/Remy & Terese (AW) 2 p.m. Make Your Point (AA) 3:30 p.m. One-on-One In-Room Visits (AW)
6 10 a.m. Catholic Communion (CH) **Music w/Lawrence & Raymond after lunch in activity area** 2 p.m. Russian Orthodox Catholic Service (CH)	**7 SHOPPING REQUESTS DUE!!!** 9 a.m. Fun Fitness Stretches (N) 10 a.m. Horseshoes (AA) 1:30 p.m. Stamps (AK) 1:30 p.m. Have You Ever? (N) 2:30 p.m. Chimes (AA) 3:30 p.m. Sensory Stim (AW) 6 p.m. Who Dun It Puzzles (AA)	**8** 9:15 a.m. Cooking Club (AK) 9:30 a.m. Classical Music w/Joe (AA) 10 a.m. Library Cart (AW) 10:45 a.m. Morning Glory Chapel (CH) **2 p.m. Music w/Roger Ellis (AA)** 3:30 p.m. Hands Alive (AW)	**9** 9 a.m. Memories (AW) 9:45 a.m. Friends & Fellowship (CH) 10:15 a.m. Dartball Team Practice (AA) 11:45 a.m. Stretchercize (DR) 1:30 p.m. Rosary (CH) 2 p.m. Catholic Mass (CH) **2:45 p.m. Bingo w/American Legion (DR)** 4 p.m. Out to Supper Bunch (O)	**10 Golfer's Day!** 9:15 a.m. Sunshine Group (AK) **9:30 a.m. Golf Putting w/students (AA)** 10 a.m. Five Alive (AK) 2 p.m. Music w/Phil John (AA) 3:30 p.m. One-on-One Room Visits (AW)	**11 World's Largest Trivia Contest, Stevens Point, WI** **9:30 a.m. Reading Group w/McKinley 3rd Graders (DR)** 10:30 a.m. Tae kwon do (DR) **2 p.m. PCHCC Trivia Contest (AA)** 3:30 p.m. One-on-One Room Visits (AW)	**12** Weekend Trivia (AW) 9 a.m. Morning Stretch (AW) 10 a.m. Reading Group w/Anne (DR) 10 a.m. Pet Therapy w/Remy & Terese (AW) 2 p.m. Giant Crosswords (AA) 3:30 p.m. One-on-One In-Room Visits (AW)

Sunday	Monday	Tuesday	Wednesday	Thursday	Friday	Saturday
13 National Garden Week! 10 a.m. Catholic Communion (CH) **Music w/Lawrence & Raymond after lunch in activity area** 2 p.m. Russian Orthodox Catholic Service (CH)	**14 SHOPPING REQUESTS DUE!!!** 9 a.m. Fun Fitness Stretches (N) 10 a.m. Sing Along w/Louise Lane (AA) 1:30 p.m. Stamps (AK) 1:30 p.m. Imagine That! (N) 1:45 p.m. One-on-One Room Visits (E) 2:30 p.m. Chimes (AA) 3:30 p.m. Garden Sensory Stim (AW) 6 p.m. Jeopardy (AA)	**15 U.S. Income Tax Day!** 9:30 a.m. Tic Tac Toe Bean Bag (AA) 10 a.m. Library Cart (AW) 10:45 a.m. Morning Glory Chapel (CH) 2 p.m. Monthly Birthday Party (AK) 2:45 p.m. Red Hat Groovy Grannies/Master Gardener Demonstration (AA) 3:30 p.m. One-on-One Therapeutic Massage (AW)	**16** 9 a.m. Memories (AW) 9:45 a.m. Friends & Fellowship (CH) 10:15 a.m. Canaland Day Care Visits (AA) 11:45 a.m. Stretchersize (DR) 1:30 p.m. Rosary (CH) 2 p.m. Catholic Mass (CH) **2:30 p.m. Music w/David, Chet & Gang (AA)** 6 p.m. Card Club (AA)	**17** 9:15 a.m. Sunshine Group (AK) **9:30 a.m. Bowling w/students (AA)** 10 a.m. Mothballs in My Attic (AK) **2 p.m. Music w/Jim Vollmer (AA)** 3:30 p.m. One-on-One Room Visits (AW)	**18** 9 a.m. Morning Greeting (N) 10 a.m. Big Ball Fun (AA) 1:30 p.m. Country Bus Ride (O) 2 p.m. Reminisce Board Game (AK) 3:30 p.m. One-on-One Room/Sensory Garden Visits (AW) 4:30 p.m. Music w/Marilyn Pederson (AA)	**19** Weekend Trivia (AW) 9 a.m. Morning Stretch (AW) 10 a.m. Scrapbooking (AK) 10 a.m. Pet Therapy w/Remy & Terese (AW) 2 p.m. Spin the Bottle (AA) 3:30 p.m. Patio Visits/Reminiscing/Activity Patio
20 National Wildlife Week! National Park Week! 10 a.m. Catholic Communion (CH) **Music w/Lawrence & Raymond after lunch in activity area** 2 p.m. Russian Orthodox Catholic Service (CH)	**21 SHOPPING REQUESTS DUE!!!** 9 a.m. Fun Fitness Stretches (N) 10 a.m. Imagination Book Fair (AA) 10 – 2 1:30 p.m. Spring Things Picture Set (N) 1:30 p.m. One-on-One Reading (E) 2:30 p.m. Resident Council Steering Committee (AK) 3:30 p.m. Spring/Garden Sensory Stim (AW) 6 p.m. Fun with Wii (AA)	**22 Earth Day!** 9:30 a.m. Classical Music w/Joe (AA) 10 a.m. Library Cart (AW) 10:45 a.m. Morning Glory Chapel (CH) **11:30 a.m. Annual Volunteer Recognition (DR)** 2 p.m. Price Is Right Board Game (AK) 3:30 Hands Alive (AW)	**23** 9 a.m. Memories (AW) 9:45 a.m. Friends & Fellowship (CH) 10:15 a.m. Dartball Team Practice (AA) 11:45 a.m. Stretchersize (DR) 1:30 p.m. Rosary (CH) 2 p.m. Catholic Mass (CH) 2:30 p.m. Social Time (DR) 3:30 p.m. Card Club (AA) 6 p.m. Casino Bingo (DR)	**24** 9:15 a.m. Sunshine Group (AK) **9:30 a.m. Jarts w/students (AA)** 10 a.m. Five Alive (AK) 2 p.m. Clem's Music Makers (AA) 3:30 p.m. One-on-One Room Visits (AW)	**25 National Arbor Day! National Hairstylist Appreciation Day!** 9 a.m. Morning Greeting (N) 10 a.m. Yoga (AA) 2 p.m. Arbor Day and Spring Slide Show (AA) 3:30 p.m. One-on-One Room/Sensory Garden Visits (AW)	**26** Weekend Trivia (AW) 9 a.m. Morning Stretch (AW) 10 a.m. Reading Group w/Anne (DR) 10 a.m. Pet Therapy w/Remy & Terese (AW) 2 p.m. The Rhythm Airs Polka Show (AA) 3:30 p.m. Patio Visits/Reminiscing/Activity Patio
27 National Volunteer Week! 10 a.m. Catholic Communion (CH) **Music w/Lawrence & Raymond after lunch in activity area** 2 p.m. Russian Orthodox Catholic Service (CH)	**28 SHOPPING REQUESTS DUE!!!** 9 a.m. Fun Fitness Stretches (N) 10 a.m. Singalong w/Alice & Friends (AA) 1:30 p.m. Stamps (AK) 1:30 p.m. Shut the Box (N) 1:30 p.m. One-on-One Reading/Trivia (E) 2:30 p.m. Chimes (AA) 3:30 p.m. Spring Sensory Stim (AW) 4 p.m. Casino Trip & Out to Supper (O)	**29** 9:15 a.m. Cooking Club (AK) 9:30 a.m. Classical Music w/Joe (AA) 10 a.m. Library Cart (AW) 10:45 a.m. Morning Glory Chapel (CH) 2 p.m. Match Game (DR) 3:30 p.m. One-on-One Therapeutic Massage (AW)	**30** 9 a.m. Memories (AW) 9:45 a.m. Friends & Fellowship (CH) 10:15 a.m. Dartball Team Practice (AA) 11:45 a.m. Stretchersize (DR) 1:30 p.m. Rosary (CH) 2 p.m. Catholic Mass (CH) 2:30 p.m. Movie & Popcorn (AA) 6 p.m. Card Club (AA)			

*Please note: Daily crosswords are available in the activity area for pickup on Mon. Tues. Wed. & Thur. Check main activity board for answers the following day.

Spring

APRIL 2008 SPECIALIZED PROGRAMMING/
SOUTH PORTAGE COUNTY HEALTH CARE CENTER

ACTIVITIES DIRECTOR: DEBBIE BERA
ACTIVITIES ASSISTANTS: MIRA MELCHER(EAST/SOUTH) TINA BERG(SOUTH)

SCHEDULE SUBJECT TO CHANGE/OBSERVE DAILY POSTINGS

CODE
AA = Activity Area
AK = Activity Kitchen
AW = All Wings
CH = Chapel
O = Outing

SR = Sensory Room
DR = Dining Room
E = East Wing
N = North Wing
S = South Wing
FR = Family Room

SUNDAY	MONDAY	TUESDAY	WEDNESDAY	THURSDAY	FRIDAY	SATURDAY
		1 National Fun At Work Day! April Fool's Day! 9:30 a.m. Ring Toss (AA) 10:45 a.m. Morning Glory Chapel (CH) 2 p.m. Shake Loose a Memory (AK) 3:30 p.m. One-on-One Therapeutic Massage (AW) 6 p.m. Rec Game/Creative Expression (S) 6:30 p.m. Let's Relax: Massage, Aromatherapy, Sensory (SR) 7 p.m. Story Hour/Reminiscing (SR)	**2** 9 a.m. Memories (AW) 9:45 a.m. Friends & Fellowship (CH) 11:45 a.m. Stretchercize (DR) 1:30 p.m. Rosary (CH) 2 p.m. Catholic Mass (CH) **2:30 p.m. Music w/David, Chet & Gang (AA)** 6 p.m. Rec Game/Creative Expression (S) 6:30 p.m. Let's Relax: Massage, Aromatherapy, Sensory (SR) 7 p.m. Story Hour/Reminiscing (SR)	**3** 9:15 a.m. Sunshine Group (AK) **9:30 a.m. Disc Golf w/students (AA)** 10:30 a.m. Church of the Intercession and Holy Communion (CH) 2 p.m. Music w/Gene Hersey (AA) 3:30 p.m. Spinner Game (S) 6 p.m. Rec Game/Creative Expression (S) 6:30 p.m. Let's Relax: Massage, Aromatherapy, Sensory (SR) 7 p.m. Story Hour/Reminiscing (SR)	**4** 9:15 a.m. Everyday Objects (S) 10 a.m. Pilates (AA) **1:30 p.m. CDA Bingo (DR)** 3:30 p.m. Multisensory Room Programs (S) 4:30 p.m. Music w/Marilyn Pederson (AA) 6 p.m. Rec Game/Creative Expression (S) 6:30 p.m. Let's Relax: Massage, Aromatherapy, Sensory (SR) 7 p.m. Story Hour/Reminiscing (SR)	**5** 8:30 a.m. Multisensory Room Programs (S) 9 a.m. Morning Stretch (AW) 10 a.m. Busy Bee Crafts (AK) 10 a.m. Reading Group w/Anne (DR) 10 a.m. Pet Therapy w/Remy & Terese (AW) 3:30 p.m. Multisensory Room Programs (S)
6 8:30 a.m. Multisensory Room Programs (S) 10 a.m. Catholic Communion (CH) **Music w/Lawrence & Raymond after lunch in activity area** 2 p.m. Russian Orthodox Catholic Service (CH) 3:30 p.m. Multisensory Room Programs (S)	**7** 9:15 a.m. Creative Writing (S) 10 a.m. Horseshoes (AA) 1:30 p.m. Color Dominoes (S) 3:30 p.m. Sensory Stim (AW) 6 p.m. Rec Game/Creative Expression (S) 6:30 p.m. Let's Relax: Massage, Aromatherapy, Sensory (SR) 7 p.m. Story Hour/Reminiscing (SR)	**8** 9:30 a.m. Classical Music w/Joe (AA) 10:45 a.m. Morning Glory Chapel (CH) **2 p.m. Music w/Roger Ellis (AA)** 3:30 p.m. Hands Alive (AW) 6 p.m. Rec Game/Creative Expression (S) 6:30 p.m. Let's Relax: Massage, Aromatherapy, Sensory (SR) 7 p.m. Story Hour/Reminiscing (SR)	**9** 9 a.m. Memories (AW) 9:45 a.m. Friends & Fellowship (CH) 11:45 a.m. Stretchercize (DR) 1:30 p.m. Rosary (CH) 2 p.m. Catholic Mass (CH) **2:45 p.m. Bingo w/American Legion (DR)** 6 p.m. Rec Game/Creative Expression (S) 6:30 p.m. Let's Relax: Massage, Aromatherapy, Sensory (SR) 7 p.m. Story Hour/Reminiscing (SR)	**10** Golfer's Day! 9:15 a.m. Sunshine Group (AK) **9:30 a.m. Golf Putting w/students (AA)** 10 a.m. Five Alive (AK) 2 p.m. Music w/Phil John (AA) 3:30 p.m. Do You Recall? (S) 6 p.m. Rec Game/Creative Expression (S) 6:30 p.m. Let's Relax: Massage, Aromatherapy, Sensory (SR) 7 p.m. Story Hour/Reminiscing (SR)	**11** World's Largest Trivia Contest, Stevens Point, WI 9:15 a.m. Grandma's Attic Bingo (S) **9:30 a.m. Reading Group w/McKinley 3rd Graders (DR)** 10:30 a.m. Tae kwon do (DR) **2 p.m. PCHCC Trivia Contest (AA)** 3:30 p.m. Multisensory Room Programs (S) 6 p.m. Rec Game/Creative Expression (S) 6:30 p.m. Let's Relax: Massage, Aromatherapy, Sensory (SR) 7 p.m. Story Hour/Reminiscing (SR)	**12** 8:30 a.m. Multisensory Room Programs (S) 9 a.m. Morning Stretch (AW) 10 a.m. Reading Group w/Anne (DR) 10 a.m. Pet Therapy w/Remy & Terese (AW) 2 p.m. Giant Crosswords (AA) 3:30 p.m. Multisensory Room Programs (S)

13 National Garden Week!
8:30 a.m. Multisensory Room Programs (S)
10 a.m. Catholic Communion (CH)
Music w/Lawrence & Raymond after lunch in activity area
2 p.m. Russian Orthodox Catholic Service (CH)
3:30 p.m. Multisensory Room Programs (S)

14
9:15 a.m. Music w/Movement (S)
10 a.m. Sing Along w/Louise Lane (AA)
1:30 p.m. Memory Matching (S)
3:30 p.m. Garden Sensory Stim (AW)
6 p.m. Rec Game/Creative Expression (S)
6:30 p.m. Let's Relax: Massage, Aromatherapy, Sensory (SR)
7 p.m. Story Hour/Reminiscing (SR)

15 U.S. Income Tax Day!
9:30 a.m. Tic Tac Toe Bean Bag (AA)
10:45 a.m. Morning Glory Chapel (CH)
2 p.m. Monthly Birthday Party (AK)
3:30 p.m. 1:1 Therapeutic Massage (AW)
6 p.m. Rec Game/Creative Expression (S)
6:30 p.m. Let's Relax: Massage, Aromatherapy, Sensory (SR)
7 p.m. Story Hour/Reminiscing (SR)

16
9 a.m. Memories (AW)
9:45 a.m. Friends & Fellowship (CH)
10:15 a.m. Canaland Day Care Visits (AA)
11:45 a.m. Stretchersize (DR)
1:30 p.m. Rosary (CH)
2 p.m. Catholic Mass (CH)
2:30 p.m. Music w/David, Chet & Gang (AA)
6 p.m. Rec Game/Creative Expression (S)
6:30 p.m. Let's Relax: Massage, Aromatherapy, Sensory (SR)
7 p.m. Story Hour/Reminiscing (SR)

17
9:15 a.m. Sunshine Group (AK)
9:30 a.m. Bowling w/students (AA)
10 a.m. Mothballs in My Attic (AK)
2 p.m. Music w/Jim Vollmer (AA)
3:30 p.m. Hidden Treasures (S)
6 p.m. Rec Game/Creative Expression (S)
6:30 p.m. Let's Relax: Massage, Aromatherapy, Sensory (SR)
7 p.m. Story Hour/Reminiscing (SR)

18
9:15 a.m. Memory Squared (S)
10 a.m. Big Ball Fun (AA)
1:30 p.m. Country Bus Ride (O)
2 p.m. Reminisce Board Game (AK)
3:30 p.m. One-on-One Room/Sensory Garden Visits (AW)
4:30 p.m. Music w/Marilyn Pederson (AA)
6 p.m. Rec Game/Creative Expression (S)
6:30 p.m. Let's Relax: Massage, Aromatherapy, Sensory (SR)
7 p.m. Story Hour/Reminiscing (SR)

19
8:30 a.m. Multisensory Room Programs (S)
9 a.m. Morning Stretch (S)
10 a.m. Reading Group w/Anne (DR)
10 a.m. Pet Therapy w/Remy & Terese (AW)
2 p.m. Spin the Bottle (AA)
3:30 p.m. Multisensory Room Programs (S)
3:30 p.m. Patio Visits/Reminiscing/Activity Patio

20 National Wildlife Week! National Park Week!
8:30 a.m. Multisensory Room Programs (S)
10 a.m. Catholic Communion (CH)
Music w/Lawrence & Raymond after lunch in activity area
2 p.m. Russian Orthodox Catholic Service (CH)
3:30 p.m. Multisensory Room Programs (S)

21
9:15 a.m. Noodle Ball & Noodle Exercise (S)
10 a.m. Imagination Book Fair (AA)
10 – 2
1:30 p.m. Dice Game (S)
3:30 p.m. Spring Garden Sensory Stim (AW)
6 p.m. Rec Game/Creative Expression (S)
6:30 p.m. Let's Relax: Massage, Aromatherapy, Sensory (SR)
7 p.m. Story Hour/Reminiscing (SR)

22 Earth Day!
9:30 a.m. Classical Music w/Joe (AA)
10:45 a.m. Morning Glory Chapel (CH)
2 p.m. One-on-One Sensory Stim (S)
3:30 p.m. Hands Alive (AW)
6 p.m. Rec Game/Creative Expression (S)
6:30 p.m. Let's Relax: Massage, Aromatherapy, Sensory (SR)
7 p.m. Story Hour/Reminiscing (SR)

23
9 a.m. Memories (AW)
9:45 a.m. Friends & Fellowship (CH)
11:45 a.m. Stretchersize (DR)
1:30 p.m. Rosary (CH)
2 p.m. Catholic Mass (CH)
2:30 p.m. Social Time (DR)
6 p.m. Rec Game/Creative Expression (S)
6:30 p.m. Let's Relax: Massage, Aromatherapy, Sensory (SR)
7 p.m. Story Hour/Reminiscing (SR)

24
9:15 a.m. Sunshine Group (AK)
9:30 a.m. Jarts w/students (AA)
10 a.m. Five Alive (AK)
2 p.m. Clem's Music Makers (AA)
3:30 p.m. One-on-One Room/Sensory Garden Visits (AW)
6 p.m. Rec Game/Creative Expression (S)
6:30 p.m. Let's Relax: Massage, Aromatherapy, Sensory (SR)
7 p.m. Story Hour/Reminiscing (SR)

25 National Arbor Day! National Hairstylist Appreciation Day!
9:15 a.m. Name 5 (S)
10 a.m. Yoga (AA)
2 p.m. Arbor Day and Spring Slide Show (AA)
3:30 p.m. One-on-One Room/Sensory Garden Visits (AW)
6 p.m. Rec Game/Creative Expression (S)
6:30 p.m. Let's Relax: Massage, Aromatherapy, Sensory (SR)
7 p.m. Story Hour/Reminiscing (SR)

26
8:30 a.m. Multi sensory Room Programs(S)
9 a.m. Morning Stretch(AW)
10 a.m. Reading Group w/Anne (DR)
10 a.m. Pet Therapy w/Remy & Terese(AW)
2 p.m. The Rhythm Airs Polka Show(AA)
3:30 p.m. Multi Sensory Room Programs(S)
3:30 p.m. Patio Visits/Reminiscing/Activity Patio

27 National Volunteer Week!
8:30 a.m. Multisensory Room Programs (S)
10 a.m. Catholic Communion (CH)
Music w/Lawrence & Raymond after lunch in activity area
2 p.m. Russian Orthodox Catholic Service (CH)
3:30 p.m. Multisensory Room Programs (S)

28
9:15 a.m. Folded Paper Paintings (S)
10 a.m. Singslong w/Alice & Friends (AA)
1:30 p.m. Dusterball (S)
3:30 p.m. Spring Sensory Stim (AW)
6 p.m. Rec Game/Creative Expression (S)
6:30 p.m. Let's Relax: Massage, Aromatherapy, Sensory (SR)
7 p.m. Story Hour/Reminiscing (SR)

29
9:30 a.m. Classical Music w/Joe (AA)
10:45 a.m. Morning Glory Chapel (CH)
2 p.m. Match Game (DR)
3:30 p.m. One-on-One Therapeutic Massage (AW)
6 p.m. Rec Game/Creative Expression (S)
6:30 p.m. Let's Relax: Massage, Aromatherapy, Sensory (SR)
7 p.m. Story Hour/Reminiscing (SR)

30
9 a.m. Memories (AW)
9:45 a.m. Friends & Fellowship (CH)
11:45 a.m. Stretchersize (DR)
1:30 p.m. Rosary (CH)
2 p.m. Catholic Mass (CH)
2:30 p.m. Movie & Popcorn (AA)
6 p.m. Rec Game/Creative Expression (S)
6:30 p.m. Let's Relax: Massage, Aromatherapy, Sensory (SR)
7 p.m. Story Hour/Reminiscing (SR)

Spring

*Please note: Multisensory room programs occur throughout the day everyday by all members of the staff, scheduled and spontaneously; before and after meals.

Chapter 12

Involving Residents and Family Members in Activities

There are two components to involving residents and family members in activities. The first is to get their input on activities that are offered. The second is to get them to participate in the activities that are offered by providing the motivation and incentive to do so.

Because an activities program is a reflection of the interests, needs, desires, and abilities of the facility's residents, it is essential for activities professionals to include residents when planning activities. There are several ways to accomplish this. A part of the Resident Council (or Resident Group) should be devoted to discussing activities that are ongoing, seeking resident input regarding what they would like to see more of, and encouraging residents to come up with ideas for new activities. Another option is to have an Activities Planning Committee composed of residents, activities staff members, family members, and other interested parties, that would meet monthly to discuss upcoming activity offerings. Incorporating a "Wishing Well" activity (loosely based on a "Make a Wish" type of activity) into your program is another way to get individual residents to suggest activities.

Activities professionals should be paying attention to the participation level (or lack of participation level) and the responses (positive and negative) to each activity that is held. This provides you with a good clue as to whether residents enjoy that particular activity and whether it is an appropriate and important part of the offerings from their perspective. A good habit to develop is to simply ask the participants how they liked a new activity and really listen to their responses. They may offer good suggestions on how to make the activity more interesting the next time.

Activities professionals should also develop relationships with family members and seek their input on activities. This can be done formally with a resident and family survey given annually as part of your continuous quality improvement (or quality assurance). It can also be done by seeking input informally from family members who participate in group activities with their loved ones. It is important that you inform family members either in casual conversation or at care plan conferences that it is important for you to have feedback on the activities that are offered. Activities professionals need to make themselves accessible to both residents and family members to address any concerns/issues and to encourage and develop relationships that foster mutual respect. After all, both activities professionals and residents' family members have the same goal: to enhance the residents' quality of life through the activities program.

Our relationships with our family members are very important to our well-being and they improve our quality of life. Activities professionals have a very important role in helping residents and their family members maintain their relationships. An easy way to do this is to encourage family members to attend activities with their loved ones. Most activities can be open to family members and the activities program should include special events that are specifically planned for large gatherings of family members and residents. These special resident/family events should promote fun, conversation, and relationships between residents and their individual families as well as peers and their families. Festive, fun events planned throughout the year guarantee happy residents and family members. Just like a mother is the "caretaker," "overseer," and "nurturer" of the home, the activities professional and activity program set the tone for the overall happiness of the nursing home. If residents/families are happy and engaged in meaningful activities, the facility is seen as a "home" where people feel accepted, connected, valued, and loved.

Use some or all of the following activities to aid you on the journey to excellence for your residents and their family members.

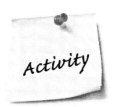

Activity — Annual Picnic

Target audience: All residents and their families, staff members, and volunteers who enjoy social opportunities, based on resident interests and needs

Objectives/outcomes:

- To promote social interactions among residents, families, and peers

- To provide an opportunity for residents and families to enjoy time spent together and to maintain and/or form new relationships/friendships

- To provide an opportunity for reminiscence

- To promote a good time enjoying the outdoors

- To promote self-esteem

Recommended group size: Large

Suggested time frame: 1.5 – 2 hours

Special needs/ability level (physical/cognitive skills needed): Can accommodate all physical and cognitive levels. Primarily a social activity.

Activity outline:

- This event involves preplanning and is a joint effort between the Dietary Department and the Activities Department.

- This is a facility-wide event and all staff members are expected to assist residents on their way out and back in, as well as help them while they are outdoors. You will also need to schedule a lot of volunteers to assist with resident transport, serving, cleanup, and so on. The Maintenance Department will have to set up and take down the event (e.g., chairs, tables, tent, etc.). The nursing staff is needed to offer assistance with eating to those who need it.

- You will need to create posters to advertise the event; you should also advertise it in the facility newsletter, activities calendar, and local newspaper. (It helps to hold this event annually in the same month, such as August as the last hurrah of summer.) You could also make invitations, but once it becomes an annual event people will expect and plan for it.

- This is an outdoor event, and you will need two serving tables, tables for residents and guests, lawn/folding chairs, lots of shade, sunscreen, hats, sunglasses, garbage cans, serving supplies and disposable dishware, outdoor extension cords for food warmers, and musicians. (Renting a large, open tent is a recommendation.) Set up everything the morning of the event or the afternoon before.

- Set up a buffet table (but have the staff serve everyone for infection control purposes); encourage residents and family members to come through the line on their own. Have staff members/volunteers available to serve residents who do not have guests.

- Menu items can include beer, soda, grilled hamburgers and bratwurst, condiments (ketchup, mustard, onions, lettuce, tomatoes, cheese, sauerkraut, etc.), potato salad, baked beans, watermelon, and ice cream bars.

- Schedule a musical entertainer to play while everyone is eating.

- Take pictures of residents and their families to remember the fun.

Helpful hints/notes: Serve residents and their families first; then serve the staff and volunteers. Observe all infection-control guidelines and individual resident dietary needs/restrictions when serving food and beverages. You must know of any food allergies your residents may have. Assemble all needed equipment and supplies prior to the start of the activity. Save all the information you've gathered for this event, laminate it or put it in plastic sleeves, and place it in a binder or folder labeled "Annual Picnic," and you now have an annual event already planned for years to come.

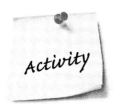

Comfort Cart

Target audience: Residents who are in the dying process and their families; also, residents who prefer to stay in their room or are confined to their room

Objectives/outcomes:

- To provide comfort and solace to residents who enter the nursing home, or who are terminally ill, confined to their room/bed for most of the day, and/or prefer to stay in their room for their personal well-being

- To offer residents, families, and guests relief during difficult visits

- To offer respite in providing something to do

- To nurture residents and families based on the religious/meditative contents of the cart

- To provide the staff a means of providing support to a resident who may not have family or friends to visit

Recommended group size: One-on-one, individual in-room activity

Suggested time frame: Left in room for as long as needed

Special needs/ability level (physical/cognitive skills needed): All functioning residents

Activity outline:

- You will need to set up a cart with items for this purpose.

- The activities director organizes and leads, with the assistance of other staff members, a yearly inservice explaining the purpose and function of the Comfort Cart. The targeted audience includes, but is not limited to, CNAs and nurses. This inservice takes place in January.

- Any staff member or family member makes referrals for the Comfort Cart using the following criteria:

– Newly admitted residents with a terminal diagnosis

– A current resident who is terminal, is room-bound, or prefers the comfort of his or her room to meet his or her psychosocial needs

– Such residents who do not have a TV, tape/CD player, and/or materials as provided on the Comfort Cart that offer solace and leisure

• You should store the Comfort Cart in a location where all staff members can access it 24/7. Upon receiving a referral, the staff member checks out the Comfort Cart, delivers and sets up the Comfort Cart in the resident's room, and instructs the unit staff members and family members on its use. The Activities Department maintains a checkout system to identify the whereabouts of the Comfort Cart at all times.

• The activities and/or social services staff checks with the unit staff, the resident, and family members to ensure continued appropriate use of the Comfort Cart to meet the resident's and/or family's needs. The cart remains in the resident's room as long as it meets the needs of the resident and/or family, or until the resident dies.

• The staff returns the Comfort Cart to its proper location when it is no longer needed and checks the cart back in on the log sheet.

• The staff inventories the contents of the Comfort Cart after each use. Missing and/or damaged items are reported to the Activities Department and are repaired or replaced as needed.

• The staff member who returned the Comfort Cart after use checks to ensure that it is clean and orderly, so it is functional for the next use.

• The Activities Department accepts donations, such as gifts of money and/or materials to be added to the contents of the Comfort Cart, at any time. Material donations should include videos, DVDs, reading materials, and CDs and/or cassette tapes that span a variety of religious beliefs or that offer respite and solace for the resident(s).

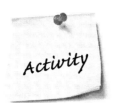

Activity | **Craft and Bake Sale**

Target audience: All residents and their families

Objectives/outcomes:

- To provide an opportunity to fundraise for activity needs outside the scope of the Activities Department's budget

- To provide an opportunity for residents and families to shop and support the cause

- To provide an opportunity for residents and families to volunteer

- To promote social interactions among residents, families, and peers

- To provide an opportunity for residents and families to enjoy time spent together and to maintain and/or form new relationships/friendships

- To get residents and their families into the holiday spirit

Recommended group size: Residents and families visit and flow through throughout the day.

Suggested time frame: 5 – 6 hours

Special needs/ability level (physical/cognitive skills needed): Primarily for residents with moderate to high functioning, though low-functioning residents enjoy looking around and observing what is going on.

Activity outline:

- Hold this event annually prior to the holidays, in October or November. This can be your official kick-off holiday event.

- Six to eight weeks prior to the event, post a sign-up sheet for residents, staff members, family members, and volunteers to sign up as vendors for selling crafts or baked goods.

- Advertise in the community for vendors as well. Keep a list of names and contact numbers to use from year to year.

- About three weeks prior to the event, mail letters to families and volunteers seeking donations and help with the event. (Eventually, they will come to expect and look for this letter.)

- Vendors reserve a table (8 ft.), with no upfront fee. Vendors pay 10% of their total sales at the end of the day to the Activities Department (alternatively, you can use whatever system would work best for your facility). If space allows, some vendors may reserve more tables. You will need to secure tables and folding chairs for this event as well.

- Have your resident craft groups make crafts throughout the year to sell at this event. Residents may also sell personal craft items by reserving their own table. Secure volunteers or family members to assist them.

- During the two weeks leading up to the event, schedule baking groups for residents to bake items that will sell well. (Freeze them to keep them fresh.) You can also seek donated baked goods as well.

- Have your Dietary Department bake fresh cinnamon rolls (often, your food vendor will donate items) for morning sales and fresh bread for afternoon sales as their contribution to the event.

- Solicit donated items for a raffle as well, and have your Resident Council sell raffle tickets the day of the event. (Make sure you have any necessary raffle license.)

- Purchase a good brand of frozen pizza in bulk and make and sell pizza over the lunch hour, particularly to the vendors, but have enough on hand for residents, families, volunteers, and staff members to purchase by the slice as well.

- As a courtesy to vendors and visitors alike, offer free hot coffee.

- Have volunteers on hand to assist with the many tasks.

- Have entertainers scheduled to play holiday background music or play holiday background music on CDs.

- Have the Resident Council decide how to use the profits from the Craft and Bake Sale. (Some ideas include purchasing a wheelchair-accessible swing, a Disklavier piano, a bird aviary, multisensory room supplies—any big-ticket item that is outside the scope of your budget.)

Variations/adaptations/modifications: You can sell any kind of treat or food item that you think would be a good seller (e.g., soup, chili, slices of pie with ice cream, cheesecake by the slice, etc.).

Helpful hints/notes: Attempt to get many of the items donated or sponsored by local businesses. Observe all infection-control guidelines and individual resident dietary needs/restrictions when serving food and beverages. You must know of any food allergies your residents may have. Assemble all needed equipment and supplies prior to the start of the activity. Save all the information you've gathered for this event, laminate it or put it in plastic sleeves, and place it in a binder or folder labeled "Craft and Bake Sale," and you now have an annual event already planned for years to come.

Facility Dog Show

Target audience: All residents and their families, staff members, and volunteers who enjoy animals and social opportunities, based on resident interests and needs

Objectives/outcomes:

- To promote social interactions among residents, families, and peers

- To provide an opportunity for residents and families to enjoy time spent together and to maintain and/or form new relationships/friendships

- To provide an opportunity for reminiscence

- To promote relationships between residents and animals

- To promote self-esteem

Recommended group size: Large

Suggested time frame: One hour

Special needs/ability level (physical/cognitive skills needed): Can accommodate all physical and cognitive levels. Primarily a social activity.

Activity outline:

- This event involves preplanning and is a joint effort between the Activities Department and all staff members.

- You need to create posters to advertise the event; you can also advertise it in the facility newsletter and put it on the activities calendar. (It helps to hold the event annually in the same month, such as April as a spring event.)

- You will need a sign-up poster for staff members, family members, and residents to sign up.

- Dogs and owners should "strut" their stuff on a "carpeted runaway" with audience members sitting on both sides. Dogs should perform tricks as directed by their owners.

- Award participation certificates (or ribbons) to dogs and their owners. You could also create certificates for Best in Show, Best Behaved, Cutest, Most Obedient , etc., and have residents be the judges.

- Have "doggie" treats in goody bags to give out to the dogs after the show. Residents can prepare them ahead of time as a helping activity. You also can schedule a "doggie biscuit" baking group as another preactivity to this event.

- Allow the audience, dog owners, and dogs some interaction (petting) time after the official show.

- Take pictures of residents and their families to remember the fun.

Helpful hints/notes: Plan ahead for "doggie accidents" by having gloves, old towels, and other such items on hand. Assemble all needed equipment and supplies prior to the start of the activity. Save all the information you've gathered for this event, laminate it or put it in plastic sleeves, and place it in a binder or folder labeled "Annual Dog Show," and you now have an annual event already planned for years to come.

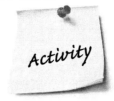

Activity | **Father's Day Brunch**

Target audience: Male residents and their children who enjoy social opportunities, based on resident interests and needs

Objectives/outcomes:

- To promote social interactions among residents, their children, and peers

- To provide an opportunity for residents and families to enjoy time spent together and to maintain and/or form new relationships/friendships

- To provide an opportunity for reminiscence

- To provide for recognition of achievements

- To promote self-esteem

Recommended group size: Large

Suggested time frame: Two hours, so residents and families can flow in and out and so that all can be accommodated

Special needs/ability level (physical/cognitive skills needed): Can accommodate all physical and cognitive levels. Primarily a social activity.

Activity outline:

- This event involves preplanning and is a joint effort between the Dietary Department and the Activities Department.

- You need to create invitations and mail them to all male residents' families. (Mail them to the primary contact and inform him or her that he or she will need to inform other children in the family.) Schedule this as a morning activity.

- Require an RSVP so that adequate refreshments can be planned, but plan on additional attendees as not everyone will RSVP.

- The day of the event provide the nursing staff with a list of residents who had families

RSVP so that they can be ready in time for the event. All residents should be in their "Sunday best" as other families will show up unannounced.

- Set up a buffet table (but have the staff serve for infection control purposes); encourage residents and their families to come through the line on their own. Have staff members/volunteers available to serve residents who do not have guests.

- Suggested menu items include punch, coffee, hot tea, a baked egg dish or scrambled eggs, cheese, sausage and crackers, hot meatballs, crab puffs, mini wraps, baklava, coffeecake, kringles, a variety of bars, mini muffins, a fresh fruit bowl, deviled eggs, pickled herring, and smoked salmon.

- Play soft background music or have a musician play soft background music.

- Take pictures of the residents and their children. Keep one for display and give one to each resident.

Variations/adaptations/modifications: You may want to give out a boutonnière to each male resident (even if he did not have children). You could have a Father's Day Dance in the afternoon with entertainment/a band and serve lighter refreshments.

Helpful hints/notes: Decorate the dining and activity areas in a summer theme. Observe all infection-control guidelines and individual resident dietary needs/restrictions when serving food and beverages. You must know of any food allergies your residents may have. Assemble all needed equipment and supplies prior to the start of the activity. Save all the information you've gathered for this event, laminate it or put it in plastic sleeves, and place it in a binder or folder labeled "Father's Day Brunch," and you now have an annual event already planned for years to come.

Fun Fair

Target audience: All residents and their families, staff members, and volunteers who enjoy social opportunities, based on resident interests and needs

Objectives/outcomes:

- To promote social interactions among residents, families, and peers

- To provide an opportunity for residents and families to enjoy time spent together and to maintain and/or form new relationships/friendships

- To provide an opportunity for reminiscence

- To promote a good time enjoying the outdoors

- To promote self-esteem

Recommended group size: Large

Suggested time frame: 90-minute time slot; residents and families can flow in and out or stay the entire time

Special needs/ability level (physical/cognitive skills needed): Can accommodate all physical and cognitive levels. Primarily a social activity.

Activity outline:

- This event involves preplanning and is a joint effort between the Dietary Department and the Activities Department. Find a civic organization or local group to host this event both financially and by providing free volunteer labor (e.g., the Lions Club).

- This is a facility-wide event and all staff members are expected to assist residents on their way out and back in, as well as help them while they are outdoors. You will also need to schedule a lot of volunteers to assist with resident transport, serving, cleanup, and so on. The Maintenance Department will need to set up and take down the event (e.g., chairs, tables, tent, etc.).

- You need to create posters to advertise the event; you also can advertise it in the facility newsletter, activities calendar, and local newspaper. (It helps to hold this event annually in the same month, such as July as a mid-summer event.)

- This is an outdoor event, and you will need two serving tables, lawn/folding chairs, lots of shade, sunscreen, hats, sunglasses, garbage cans, a popcorn machine, serving supplies and disposable dishware, outdoor extension cords for the popcorn machine, and musicians. (Renting a large open tent is a recommendation.) Set everything up the morning of the event or the afternoon before. Helium balloons tied to wheelchairs make for a festive event.

- Set up a buffet table (but have the staff serve for infection control purposes); encourage residents and their families to come through the line on their own. Have staff members/volunteers available to serve residents who do not have guests.

- Menu items can include beer, soda, fresh popped popcorn, watermelon, ice cream cones (have several flavors available), and other "fair" snacks.

- Schedule a musical entertainer or band for the event.

- Rent a dunk tank and have staff members sit inside for 30-minute increments. Staff members, residents, and family members can all try their hand at dunking someone. (Let residents be closer to the target.)

- Take pictures of residents and their families to remember the fun.

Variations/adaptations/modifications: You could set up carnival game stations (e.g., throw baseballs at milk cartons, ring a 2-liter soda bottle, drop clothespins into a milk jug, go fishing behind a curtain, pick a duck from a pool, etc.) and have prizes to give out. These are good games for any grandchildren and great-grandchildren who attend. You will need volunteers to man the booths.

Helpful hints/notes: Attempt to get many of the items donated or sponsored by local businesses. Observe all infection-control guidelines and individual resident dietary needs/restrictions when serving food and beverages. You must know of any food allergies your residents may have. Assemble all needed equipment and supplies prior to the start of the activity. Save all the information you've gathered for this event, laminate it or put it in plastic sleeves, and place it in a binder or folder labeled "Fun Fair," and you now have an annual event already planned for years to come.

Memorial Service

Target audience: Residents, families, and staff members who want to remember those who have passed away

Objectives/outcomes:

- To remember those who have passed away

- To provide a sense of peace for residents, families, and the staff

- To help residents realize that they make a difference and that they, too, will be remembered once they are no longer with us; hence, increasing their self-esteem

- To allow for expression of grief and sadness

- To celebrate and be thankful for our relationships with others

- To recognize a higher power or spirituality and to feel connected to a higher universe

- To increase faith and promote healing

Recommended group size: Large

Suggested time frame: 45 – 60 minutes

Special needs/ability level (physical/cognitive skills needed): Primarily geared toward residents with moderate to high functioning. They need to be able to understand that they are at a remembrance service for those who have passed away.

Activity outline:

- Schedule a quarterly memorial service to recognize and remember residents who have passed away. Prepare a memorial service letter or invitation to be mailed two to three weeks prior to the service to give family members time to get off from work so that they can attend. Mail to the primary contact person and encourage family members to let other family members know about the service. Include it on your activities calendar as well. Make a poster announcing the service and those you will be remembering.

- Secure someone to prepare a sermon, or prepare one yourself. We have found it best to keep the sermon nondenominational so that everyone is comfortable taking part. It should be more of a remembrance than a church service.

- Secure a musician to play guitar, organ, or piano.

- Develop and prepare a program for the service and run off enough copies for everyone in attendance. Have the sermon, readings, poems, stories, and songs coordinate.

- As part of the remembrance, announce the names of the deceased and invite families forward to receive a token of remembrance (e.g., a bookmark, cross, angel pin, whatever you decide).

- At the conclusion of the service, invite everyone to join together for conversation and light refreshments (e.g., punch and cookies or bars).

Variations/adaptations/modifications: As part of remembering residents who pass away, also set up a memorial remembrance table where you keep a Bible, a cross, a small display commemorating the resident who recently passed away (a poem with the resident's name and date of death), and a battery operated candle. This allows for immediate recognition of an individual's death, whereas the service allows for public recognition of a collective group of individuals at a later date.

Helpful hints/notes: Develop standard sermons for quarterly services. You can always adjust them by changing the readings, hymns, prayers, and altering the sermon slightly.

Mother's Day Tea Social

Target audience: Female residents and their children who enjoy social opportunities, based on resident interests and needs

Objectives/outcomes:

- To promote social interactions among residents, their children, and peers

- To provide an opportunity for residents and their families to enjoy time spent together and to maintain and/or form new relationships/friendships

- To provide an opportunity for reminiscence

- To provide for recognition of achievements

- To promote self-esteem

Recommended group size: Large

Suggested time frame: Two hours, so residents and families can flow in and out and so that everyone can be accommodated

Special needs/ability level (physical/cognitive skills needed): Can accommodate all physical and cognitive levels. Primarily a social activity.

Activity outline:

- This event involves preplanning and is a joint effort between the Dietary Department and the Activities Department. Because Mother's Day is always the Sunday that kicks off Nursing Home Week, this can be your official kick-off event for the week's worth of special events. Schedule it as a morning activity.

- You need to create invitations and mail them to all female residents' families. (Mail them to the primary contact and inform him or her that he or she will need to inform other children in the family.)

- Require an RSVP so that adequate refreshments can be planned, but plan on additional attendees as not everyone will RSVP.

- The day of the event provide the nursing staff with a list of residents who had families RSVP so that they can be ready in time for the event. All residents should be in their "Sunday best" as other families will show up unannounced.

- Set up a buffet table (but have the staff serve for infection control purposes); encourage residents and the families to come through the line on their own. Have staff members/volunteers available to serve residents who do not have guests.

- Suggested menu items include punch, coffee, hot tea, a variety of hors d'oeuvres (e.g., cheese, sausage and crackers, hot meatballs, crab puffs, and mini wraps), baklava, petit fours, coffeecake, kringles, a variety of bars, mini muffins, scones, a fresh fruit bowl, deviled eggs, pickled herring, and smoked salmon.

- Play soft background music or have a musician play soft background music.

- Take pictures of residents and their children. Keep one for display and give one to each resident.

Variations/adaptations/modifications: You may want to give out a single, long-stemmed carnation to each female resident (even if she did not have children).

Helpful hints/notes: Decorate the dining and activity areas in a spring theme. Observe all infection-control guidelines and individual resident dietary needs/restrictions when serving food and beverages. You must know of any food allergies your residents may have. Assemble all needed equipment and supplies prior to the start of the activity. Save all the information you've gathered for this event, laminate it or put it in plastic sleeves, and place it in a binder or folder labeled "Mother's Day Tea Social," and you now have an annual event already planned for years to come.

Activity | **Outdoor Campfire Night**

Target audience: All residents and their families, staff members, and volunteers who enjoy social opportunities, based on resident interests and needs

Objectives/outcomes:

- To promote social interactions among residents, families, and peers

- To provide an opportunity for residents and families to enjoy time spent together and to maintain and/or form new relationships/friendships

- To provide an opportunity for reminiscence

- To promote a good time enjoying the outdoors and to "re-experience" some camping fun

- To promote self-esteem

Recommended group size: Large

Suggested time frame: 1.5 – 2 hours

Special needs/ability level (physical/cognitive skills needed): Can accommodate all physical and cognitive levels. Primarily a social activity.

Activity outline:

- This event involves preplanning and is a joint effort between the Activities Department and the Nursing Department.

- This is a facility-wide event and all staff members are expected to assist residents on their way out and back in, as well as help them while they are outdoors. You will also need to schedule a lot of volunteers to assist with resident transport, serving, cleanup, and so on. The Maintenance Department will need to set up and take down the event (e.g., chairs, campfire ring, campfire wood, etc.).

- You need to create posters to advertise the event; you also can advertise it in the facility newsletter, activities calendar, and local newspaper. It helps to hold this event annually in the same month, such as September as a fall activity.

- You need to create invitations and mail them to all residents' families. Mail them to the primary contact and inform him or her that he or she will need to inform other children in the family.

- This is an outdoor event and you will need lawn/folding chairs, jackets and blankets (as needed), a campfire ring, bug spray, garbage cans, a popcorn machine, serving supplies and disposable dishware, and outdoor extension cords for the musician. Set everything up the afternoon of the event.

- Set up a cart with refreshment supplies. Have staff members/volunteers available to serve residents who do not have guests.

- Menu items can include fresh popped popcorn, beer, soda, and lemonade. Other items could be offered: for example, marshmallows, graham crackers, and chocolate bars for making s'mores; hotdogs (to grill over the campfire) and buns, and so on.

- Schedule a guitar entertainer to play campfire songs and have a singalong.

- Take pictures of residents and their families to remember the fun.

Helpful hints/notes: Serve residents and their families first; then serve staff members and volunteers. Observe all infection-control guidelines and individual resident dietary needs/restrictions when serving food and beverages. You must know of any food allergies your residents may have. Assemble all needed equipment and supplies prior to the start of the activity. Save all the information you've gathered for this event, laminate it or put it in plastic sleeves, and place it in a binder or folder labeled "Outdoor Campfire Night," and you now have an annual event already planned for years to come.

Resident/Family Christmas Tea Social

Target audience: All residents and their families who enjoy social opportunities, based on resident interests and needs

Objectives/outcomes:

- To promote social interactions among residents, their children, and peers

- To provide an opportunity for residents and families to enjoy time spent together and to maintain and/or form new relationships/friendships

- To provide an opportunity for reminiscence

- To provide for recognition of achievements

- To promote self-esteem

Recommended group size: Large

Suggested time frame: 90 minutes, so residents and families can flow in and out and so that everyone can be accommodated

Special needs/ability level (physical/cognitive skills needed): Can accommodate all physical and cognitive levels. Primarily a social activity.

Activity outline:

- This event involves preplanning and is a joint effort between the Dietary Department and the Activities Department. This event is offered in place of having families purchase meal tickets and join residents for dinner on Christmas Day. It is free to families. Schedule it as an afternoon activity.

- You need to create invitations and mail them to all residents' families. (Mail them to the primary contact and inform him or her that he or she will need to inform other children in the family.)

- Require an RSVP so that adequate refreshments can be planned, but plan on additional attendees as not everyone will RSVP.

- The day of the event provide the nursing staff with a list of residents who had families RSVP so that they can be ready in time for the event. All residents should be in their "Sunday best" as other families will show up unannounced.

- Set up a buffet table (but have the staff serve for infection control purposes); encourage residents and families to come through the line on their own. Have staff members/volunteers available to serve residents who do not have guests.

- Suggested menu items include punch, coffee, hot tea, a variety of hors d'oeuvres (e.g., cheese, sausage and crackers, hot meatballs, mini BBQ sausages, crab puffs, and mini wraps or mini sandwiches), baklava, petit fours, mini muffins, Christmas cookies and bars, a fresh fruit bowl, deviled eggs, pickled herring, and smoked salmon.

- Play soft background Christmas music or have a musician play soft background Christmas music.

- Take pictures of residents and their children. Keep one for display and give one to each resident.

Variations/adaptations/modifications: Have Santa stop by for a visit and/or have carolers stop by to entertain.

Helpful hints/notes: Decorate the dining and activity areas in a Christmas theme. Observe all infection-control guidelines and individual resident dietary needs/restrictions when serving food and beverages. You must know of any food allergies your residents may have. Assemble all needed equipment and supplies prior to the start of the activity. Save all the information you've gathered for this event, laminate it or put it in plastic sleeves, and place it in a binder or folder labeled "Resident/Family Christmas Tea Social," and you now have an annual event already planned for years to come.

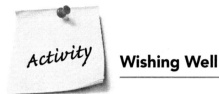

Wishing Well

Target audience: All residents

Objectives/outcomes:

- To seek input from residents (or family members if a resident is unable to express his or her thoughts) about potential new activity ideas

- To honor individual residents' "wishes"

- To encourage involvement in the development of the activities program

- To give residents a choice and a say regarding recommendations

- To increase residents' self-esteem and self-expression

- To embrace culture changes with resident-centered activities

Recommended group size: N/A, done independently

Suggested time frame: Open and available at all times

Special needs/ability level (physical/cognitive skills needed): None

Activity outline:

- Secure a "wishing well" (they can be purchased from stores where woodcrafts are sold) to keep in the activity area or in another prominent place. (The tabletop variety is good.)

- Run off "Wishing Well" forms and place them in a bin next to the "wishing well."

- Create a "Wishing Well" poster, laminate it, and place it on or next to the "wishing well."

- Advertise the activity initially with additional posters, during the Resident Council meeting and other activities, and through the facility newsletter and/or calendar.

- Incorporate suggestions into one-on-one, small-group, or large-group programs (depending on the "wish"), informing the resident how and when you are meeting his or her "wish."

- Remind residents that they can wish for any sort of activity they want, regardless of how "impossible" it might seem to them. It will be the activities professional's responsibility to figure out a way to incorporate the residents' wishes.

Helpful hints/notes: It will take much encouragement for residents to offer suggestions, as they will tend to focus on the impossibilities, their losses versus their strengths. Over time, this should become less difficult. As the culture of long-term care changes as well as the clientele (think baby boomers), the expectation will be that residents will plan the activities and the staff will be the facilitators to make sure the activities are held to meet residents' needs and expectations.

DATE DUE
